# THE ACUPUNCTURE RESPONSE

*Balance Energy and Restore Health—*
*a Western Doctor Tells You How*

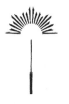

## GLENN S. ROTHFELD, M.D., M.Ac.
## and SUZANNE LEVERT

**Contemporary Books**

Chicago   New York   San Francisco   Lisbon   London   Madrid   Mexico City
Milan   New Delhi   San Juan   Seoul   Singapore   Sydney   Toronto

**Library of Congress Cataloging-in-Publication Data**

Rothfeld, Glenn S.
    The acupuncture response : balance energy and restore health : a Western doctor tells you how / Glenn S. Rothfeld and Suzanne LeVert.
        p.   cm.
    Includes index.
    ISBN 0-8092-9759-0
    1. Acupuncture.    I. LeVert, Suzanne.    II. Title.

RM184.R68    2001
615.8'92—dc21                                                2001037146

## Contemporary Books

### A Division of The McGraw·Hill Companies

    3  4  5  6  7  8  9  10    DSH/DSH    0  1  0  9  8  7  6  5

ISBN 0-8092-9759-0

This book was set in Adobe Caslon
Printed and bound by Quebecor Martinsburg

Cover and interior design by Monica Baziuk
Interior illustrations by Olivia Hartranft

McGraw-Hill books are available at special quantity discounts to use as premiums and sales promotions, or for use in corporate training programs. For more information, please write to the Director of Special Sales, Professional Publishing, McGraw-Hill, Two Penn Plaza, New York, NY 10121-2298. Or contact your local bookstore.

This book is printed on acid-free paper.

*To my patients, who teach me*
*To my family, who love me*

# CONTENTS

# ACKNOWLEDGMENTS

I THANK PROFESSOR J. R. WORSLEY for taking an ancient system of medicine and making it alive and current for his students. Five-Element acupuncture continues to be the best tool that I have in medicine. I thank my teachers over the years, including Bob Duggan, Julia Measures, Jim McCormick, Ted Kaptchuk, Robert Guillaume, Joe Helms, Tran Viet Dzung, and many others. To my acupuncture community in New England, I would like to extend my sincere appreciation of our gatherings, mutual support, and love. Thanks to Dedie, Vicki, and others whose input helped me to shape this book, and to Dan Seitz and Barbara Mitchell for their timely information. Thank you to Olivia Hartranft for her lovely illustrations.

Personally, I acknowledge my wife, Magi; my children, Emma, Carly, Jed, and Eli; my parents, always supportive and generous; and the rest of my family for their endless love and support. To Bittles, I'm sorry. Thanks to Michael Hussin, my longtime colleague and goomba. I thank my agent, Lee Ann Chearney, for her help and patience. Thanks to

Debbie Romaine for stepping in at the eleventh hour and helping us immeasurably. Finally, a special thanks to Suzanne LeVert, my coauthor. After six books together, we've developed a trust and easy working relationship that I cherish. Wonderful work, Suzanne!

PART I

# THE ART OF ACUPUNCTURE

To many Americans, the art of acupuncture is an unfamiliar one, kept to the sidelines in favor of more mainstream, Western medical techniques of diagnosis and treatment. As you'll read in this part of the book, however, the complex, elegant, and holistic nature of acupuncture—along with its proven success in treating and preventing a host of illnesses—has drawn millions of Americans to the treatment offices of acupuncturists across the country.

I

# MY JOURNEY TO ACUPUNCTURE

FOR THE PAST TWENTY YEARS, I've straddled the worlds of Western and Eastern medicine. Gradually, my work as a physician and my work as an acupuncturist have blended. From my Western training, I have learned to evaluate my patients analytically and to treat their diseases, often quite effectively depending on the condition.

From acupuncture and Chinese medicine, I've learned that we are part of the natural world and that illness can be seen as a disruption of that world. Through the eyes of this natural-healing system, I've been able to understand my patients better, not just the acupuncture patients, but all patients. I've learned that all patients come in with a story, a compilation of who they are and why they are in my office, with this particular problem, at this particular time in their lives.

I've spent the last twenty-five years discovering and mastering acupuncture and Chinese medicine, and learning to integrate these techniques into my medical practice. In many ways, my journey has mirrored the growth of acupuncture itself in the West. It is a journey that has been taken by many Americans like me. And, in the past three to four years, we've seen the reward as we near the end of that journey, as acupuncture has taken a more accepted place in the present medical system and promises to grow further in this new century. What follows is the story of my involvement with acupuncture and the concurrent growth of acupuncture in our culture.

# In the Beginning

From 1971 to 1975, I attended the State University of New York at Buffalo Medical School, at a time when the culture of the United States and other Western nations was undergoing a transformation. People of all ages, but especially those in their teens and twenties, were making an effort to return to the earth, to a more natural and peaceful way of life. The *Whole Earth Catalog* and other magazines proclaimed a new lifestyle dependent on natural foods, natural healing, and technologies that emphasized natural, organic materials.

I, too, was a product of that generation, and I entered medical school filled with a fervor to practice a different kind of medicine from the one being taught. I was deeply suspicious of the prevailing medical establishment, which I saw as too reliant on technology and drugs. At that time, the natural-healing movement was a hodgepodge of folk wisdom and cross-cultural concepts filtered through the burgeoning New Age movement. On communes and in urban centers, young people were beginning to take vitamins and herbs, learn yoga and meditation, grow food organically, and eat in a new way.

When we medical students reached our third year of training, we began treating patients, which made our learning come alive, but there was still the nagging sensation that something was missing. In effect, our whole medical training seemed to be leading to just one narrow question: "What drug should I give?" For me, steeped in the culture of the times, this question and its answer were not enough. I needed to explore the systems of natural healing that grew out of the wisdom of the ages. My medical school friends and I set about educating ourselves about new (to us) healing traditions, making up for all that our medical schools failed to teach us.

On a personal level, many of us fledgling practitioners started to change our lifestyles as well, cooking natural, organic food in woks, and stir-frying vegetables rather than cooking up a slab of meat. We read *Let's Eat Right to Keep Fit* by Adele Davis, a biochemist and nutritional writer. We even brought Davis to speak to our medical school class, and through her, I learned that B vitamins performed specific jobs in our bodies and that we, as doctors, could prescribe them to our patients in order to promote health and healing. I learned about brown rice, combining beans and grains, and the "evils" of sugar (which is still a "necessary" evil in my life!). For the first time, I made the connection between what I put in my body and how my body functioned.

And, what was more exciting to a young medical student, I discovered that the biochemistry that we were learning actually depended on vitamins, minerals, and other nutritional factors. It depended on them, but it was not taught in a way that emphasized them, so I hadn't noticed! As you'll read later in this book, teaching about diet and nutrition—and even prescribing eating plans to my patients—remains an integral part of my practice today.

When the Beatles went to India and started meditating, we started meditating as well. I learned about the studies conducted by Dr. Herbert Benson and Dr. Keith Wallace of Harvard Medical School, which showed that meditation caused beneficial physiological changes to the body—changes that could influence health and healing without the need for drugs, surgery, or other typical Western techniques. I then brought Dr. Wallace to speak to my medical school class.

An important milestone for me—and for the Western world in general—was reached while I was in my second year of medical school. In 1972, while accompanying President Richard Nixon on a state trip to China, *New York Times* columnist James Reston suffered an attack of appendicitis. To control his pain after surgery, his doctors treated him with a Chinese system of medicine called acupuncture. Reston wrote about it in the pages of the *Times*, introducing many Westerners to this system of healing.

As a medical student searching for ways to make sense of the medicine in this changing world, I was intrigued. Physicians, including one from my medical school, went to China when they learned that Chinese doctors were curing deafness with acupuncture. A dentist I knew came back from China and began to use acupuncture in his practice. On school break in New York City, I wandered into an herb store and tried to talk to the acupuncturist in the back room, but language proved too great a barrier.

Once in practice in Boston, I rekindled my interest in acupuncture, which I'd forsaken during my residency. In fact, it isn't so much that I searched for acupuncture as that acupuncture found me. It so happened that the law in Massachusetts at the time required an acupuncturist to have a supervising physician to monitor his or her practice. This was a challenge for acupuncturists, who had trouble finding physicians who had even heard of acupuncture, to say nothing of finding some who would take responsibility for them. But several local acupuncturists, knowing that I had an interest in alternative medicine, asked me to supervise their practices. Once again, I divided my time between standard medical treatments for hypertension and headaches, and the exotic (to me) world of herbs, needles, and moxibustion. (Moxibustion, the burning of an herb on an acupuncture point, is described later in the book.)

## The Needles and the Neophyte

The next step in my journey came a few years later, when a physician colleague, Dr. Paul Epstein, asked me to oversee his practice while he went to work in Mozambique. Dr. Epstein had been supervising a Chinese acupuncturist, Dr. John Shen, who practiced in a blue-collar town near Boston. Dr. Shen's office consisted of several small treatment rooms and a waiting area. Two young assistants, one Chinese and one American, followed Dr. Shen as he examined his patients.

If I expected Dr. Shen's patients to be young and oriented toward New Age practices, I was mistaken. The first patient was a burly middle-aged longshoreman who came in reporting problems of coughing and poor breathing. He had taken the medications that I would have prescribed, but he was in search of another way of treatment. Dr. Shen appraised the man's appearance, felt his pulse, and studied his tongue. (The tongue and pulse are discussed in Chapter 4.) He looked at the man and said, "Too much cold."

The American assistant explained to me that cold wind is viewed as a cause of disease in Chinese medicine, and the man was exposed to cold winds in the course of his outdoor work. Dr. Shen said that he would need to "remove the cold and wind" in order to heal the problem. He then did something for which I was quite unprepared. He rubbed a gel that smelled of menthol (I later learned that it was called tiger balm) on the man's back and then proceeded to take the metal cover off of the jar and rub it hard over the same area. Deep reddish-purple streaks that looked like dark welts appeared in several areas above and around the shoulder blades. I came to learn that this technique is called *guasha* and that this therapy, along with a technique called cupping, was used by many practitioners of Chinese medicine to resolve cold injury to the muscles.

After inserting stainless steel needles that varied from half an inch to two inches in length into the man's wrists, back, and arms, Dr. Shen moved on to the next person, a woman in her forties suffering from chronic back pain, who had been coming to the office for some time. While Dr. Shen concentrated on feeling her pulse, the patient told me about how these acupuncture treatments had enabled her to get back to work.

I listened and watched. Not knowing that there are six pulses on each side of the body and that practitioners of Chinese medicine arrive at their diagnoses largely by feeling the pulse, I was puzzled about the care and the time Dr. Shen spent in a meditative state while doing so. I watched as the doctor placed needles on points on her hands, feet, and back and then returned to the first patient to heat up the points on his back with a sweet-smelling burning herb called moxa.

I came away from this experience with a feeling of having walked into another universe. Burning herbs? Rubbing menthol gel with a jar lid? Cold wind? Twelve pulses? Mostly, I felt the enormous gulf between what I had experienced as Chinese medicine and what I had spent the last six years of my life studying. Dr. Shen's American assistant felt this gulf as well. He had been following the master around for several months but had very few of his questions answered. In Western fashion, he frequently interrupted Dr. Shen to ask something, and he was rarely rewarded with an answer. The Chinese assistant quietly moved about to retrieve needles, moxa, and tiger balm for his teacher and was given a few words of explanation between patients.

## Teaching the East in the West

In the East, most Chinese practitioners learn their art, craft, and science through apprenticeships, not organized medical schools as we do here. Unfortunately, this tradition has led to some difficulties in developing educational models in the United States. Our culture is an impatient one. Many practitioners and laypeople alike who are interested in "alternative medicine" in general tend to study yoga one year, meditation the next, *tai chi chuan* the next. We Westerners tend to get impatient when the mastery of one technique does not develop or when results from our efforts are not immediate.

As for acupuncture specifically, the first Western acupuncturists embraced the early holistic movement either because Chinese medicine's emphasis on "natural" "holistic" healing appealed to them or they were drawn to Eastern spiritual systems such as Zen or Buddhism. In these spiritual pursuits, it was common to patiently follow the master, gleaning what they could from the master's behavior until one day they realized what was being taught and became enlightened. Like a trade apprentice (acupuncture was taught like any other trade in Asia), the acupuncture student was expected to work for the teacher, who would bestow periodic instruction in return.

The first acupuncture schools founded in the United States were early attempts to merge an apprentice method with a training that was familiar to Western students. The schools, such as the New England School of Acupuncture (NESA) in Massachusetts and the Institute of Taoist Studies in Los Angeles, were built around the teachings of a master (Dr. James So at NESA; Ju Gim Shek in California), and the instructors were frequently the master's students. These training programs were not generally rigorous, certainly not by medical school terms. Many students had no college degrees. Testing was variable, and there was no exposure to Western science in general, nor to medicine specifically. At the same time, there was little awareness of acupuncture in the medical mainstream, now that the media had moved from James Reston's appendix to other pressing issues.

In cases in which one master was not present to lead students through the learning process, confusion frequently reigned. Through my own studies, I learned that this confusion stemmed from the fact that, because Chinese medicine is a wonderful patchwork of theory developed over centuries, techniques passed within families and schools, and it focused on individual treatment protocols that worked for that clinician. Put two or more teachers who had learned from different traditions in the same training program, and their students found it difficult to resolve the contradictions.

Nevertheless, acupuncture training and awareness continued to grow throughout the United States during the 1970s. Slowly, research began to appear that laid the theoretical underpinnings of acupuncture science. An early hypothesis of how pain occurs, the Gate Control theory, seemed to explain how acupuncture might block pain. In 1976,

Dr. Bruce Pomeranz published a paper demonstrating that acupuncture released a substance called endorphin, a natural pain reliever. (Current theories of acupuncture science are discussed in Chapter 3.) Clinical studies did not appear in the U.S. literature until much later, although they were occurring in Europe by this time.

By 1980, I was supervising five Western-trained acupuncturists. One was a graduate of NESA, one of the first U.S. schools and still one of the finest. The others had trained in England with British acupuncturist J. R. Worsley. Four of them worked in an office in downtown Boston, and I too saw some patients in that office. At the same time, I continued to study nutritional and herbal medicine in my off-hours and tried out what I learned on a few patients. I soon discovered the unique benefits of this approach to health and healing by working with a certain population who had specific medical needs that Western medicine was failing to address.

# Redefining "Standard Care"

My main practice consisted of a home-care program in East Boston that involved treating elderly Italian patients who lived in three-floor walk-ups in this working-class neighborhood. I discovered that, by and large, my patients were from farms and rural towns, where health care consisted of herbs, poultices, and even cupping, a process of covering the body with glass cups that are heated to create a vacuum inside. (Cupping is not unique to the Chinese culture; my grandmother came from Eastern Europe with her bag of glass cups, which she called "bankes" and which still sit on my office shelf.) Italian *camomila* (chamomile) was used to help them sleep; mustard plasters lowered their fevers; and when all else failed, some wine pressed from the grapes growing in the back-yards behind their three-floor apartments would relax their tightened muscles. I ended many days in patients' homes sharing a glass of home-made wine, sometimes with a fresh *pizelle* (Italian cookie). One elderly man, who lived alone, had had his voice box removed and was unable to talk. Once each month, I would visit him last and he would make two cups of espresso with a strong shot of anisette, a licorice-flavored liquor, which we would drink together in silence, occasionally murmuring our approval to one another.

Prescription medications were a big problem in this population. Elderly people frequently have more difficulty with digestion, and putting several different kinds of pills into the stomach can cause distress. In addition, compliance is always uncertain when it comes to taking more than one pill a day, particularly in a population that grew up taking herbs grown in the Sicilian countryside. Even reading the labels and opening the jars can be an impediment for people in their senior years. In fact, I was able to solve the problem of heart failure in one patient just by changing the lightbulb over her kitchen sink so that she could see her pill list properly! The next day, she was able to take all of the scheduled doses of her diuretic and heart medicines, and within the week, her breathing was better and her legs were less swollen.

Another of my patients had breast cancer that had spread to the bone. One day, she shifted in bed and suffered a painful fracture of the arm. She was already on heavy doses of narcotics to treat the pain caused by the cancer, so making her feel comfortable posed quite a challenge. In desperation, I called a friend, Ted Kaptchuk. Ted had trained in Chinese medicine in Macao, China, and was teaching at NESA in nearby Watertown. He and an assistant, Joyce Singer, came to the house and treated my patient with acupuncture. To my surprise, we were able to halve her medication within days.

I then realized how useful acupuncture could be to other patients in my practice, even—or perhaps especially—men and women in this population. Soon I was bringing other acupuncturists into my patients' homes, often with the same remarkable results. They treated pain, constipation, and headaches. The nurse-practitioner who assisted me took herbal prescriptions, often written in Chinese, to Chinatown and would return with strange mixtures of roots, seeds, dried fruits, and other herbs. We would cook the herbs in the patient's home and feed the concoction to the patient. To an Italian grandmother in her nineties, the smell of fresh herbs boiling frequently made more sense than the little pills we were having her swallow!

Working in the downtown Boston office, I was exposed to many satisfied acupuncture patients and to their success stories. I saw a person with once crippling arthritis able to leave the wheelchair behind. I saw another with chronic sinus infections able to avoid antibiotics after beginning treatment. I asked many patients why they came, and words such as "balance," "well-being," and "energy" were frequent responses. I still, however, hadn't experienced treatment myself.

# Physician, Heal Thyself

I had my first acupuncture treatment in 1982. I was newly separated, with two young children, and beginning to feel an incongruity between the medicine I practiced and the new ideas of healing that I was studying. I was anxious, sleepless, and in emotional pain. I turned to a friend and colleague, an acupuncturist named Jim McCormick. My first treatment consisted of having needles puncture my feet, then being left alone to nap. (I've since come to know that falling asleep during an acupuncture treatment is relatively common.) I had a dream of a tree, sprouting from the ground, with leaves just budding.

When I awoke, not ten minutes later, I felt refreshed and as if something had been released in me. Jim explained that he placed the needles where he did in order to address an energy he called the wood energy. (You'll read more about wood and other aspects of the Five-Element theory later in the book.) The wood energy involves a vision of the future, and the treatment had released some of the anger and frustration that blocked my ability to move on with my life. Having been thus exposed to the power of acupuncture, I enrolled at the Traditional Acupuncture Institute (TAI) in Columbia, Maryland, in 1983.

During my two years at TAI, I was exposed to the contradictions that are the essence of Chinese medicine. Bob Duggan, the school's director, asked us to hold seemingly opposite concepts in our heads at once, learn to juggle them, and see them as patterns rather than problems to solve. I learned that the theories that make up Chinese medicine had been woven into a patchwork quilt over the centuries, so that individual pieces reflected the thinking of specific generations and eras. This process of creating a medical tradition differs markedly from the way Western medicine developed and continues to develop. Here, we tend to give much more value to the "new" and discard the old. For example, several studies supporting the use of oat bran to lower cholesterol are negated by the latest study that does not show the exact same result. A study questioning the effects of vitamin C brings into question a whole body of work that is supportive of its use but may not have been done yesterday. The difference between the two medical systems is much like the difference between the Eastern and Western cultures, the former honoring and sometimes deifying its elders, the latter valuing youth above all other concerns.

I began to practice acupuncture in my downtown office and also continued my studies in England at the College of Traditional Chinese Acupuncture in Leamington Spa, Warwickshire. There, I was taught by Professor J. R. Worsley, who had synthesized the system now known as Five-Element acupuncture from the teachings of his instructors in England, France, and the East.

Professor Worsley wrote very little about this system. When asked how we were to study and learn, he implored us to spend time in nature every day. "Chinese medicine follows natural laws," he said. Intrinsic to all of holistic medicine is the concept of forces of nature working toward healing and health. In older texts, this is called vitalism. There, in Chinese medical theory, was a system that allowed me to actually understand the relationship between nature and illness. And I could begin to answer the question of why a patient came to the office at that moment, with that particular symptom, and how this fit into the rest of his or her life—and my own. And, with acupuncture, I could better help these patients.

# And the Movement Spreads

While I was studying in Europe and the United States, the medical acupuncture movement took off. Dr. Joe Helms, a physician from California, had developed an acupuncture training course for physicians based on the teachings of his French acupuncture professors. In France, only physicians could be acupuncturists, and the several hundred years since the Jesuits had introduced acupuncture to France had allowed a fertile medical acupuncture scene to develop. Dr. Helms's program, taught through the UCLA Medical Extension Program, began to train physicians to use acupuncture in their existing practices. Some physicians continued their training to become primarily acupuncturists; some began incorporating this new modality into their family medicine, pain management, anesthesia, and psychiatric practices. A professional organization, the American Academy of Medical Acupuncture (AAMA), was formed as an umbrella organization of physician acupuncturists and began to produce educational conferences.

Despite these advances, acupuncture rarely made it onto the radar screen of mainstream medicine. In fact, most mainstream medical doctors considered this two-thousand-year-old system new and unproven. (As Chapter 3 explains, it was unproven only by certain U.S. standards.) Then, several events triggered an expansion of acupuncture use and popularity within the medical community as well as among the population at large.

First, in 1992, the federal Food and Drug Administration took acupuncture needles off of the experimental equipment list. Prior to that time, acupuncture needles had been deemed experimental devices, and an acupuncturist technically used the needles only "for investigational purposes." The recognition that these stainless steel needles were actual tools of an accepted trade boosted acupuncture in the media and in the public's eye. New acupuncture schools were established, and state regulatory boards began to look at acupuncture as a health-care specialty. An organization called the National Commission for the Certification of Acupuncturists (now called the National Certification Commission for Acupuncture and Oriental Medicine) developed a national certification exam for acupuncturists, and states began to accept that examination as their criterion for acupuncture licensing. Another organization, the National Accreditation Commission for Schools and Colleges of Acupuncture and Oriental Medicine (now called Accreditation Commission for Acupuncture and Oriental Medicine), developed as a certifying organization for acupuncture schools. And by 1994, there were approximately eight thousand nonphysician and three thousand physician acupuncturists in the United States.

## Acupuncture for the Twenty-First Century

In 1989, I was practicing acupuncture and what was then called holistic medicine. Using the techniques that I had studied in acupuncture school and learned from conferences and training sessions, I treated patients with acupuncture for a wide variety of problems, from arthritis to depression to the side effects of chemotherapy. I began teaching at the New England School of Acupuncture, developing a Western medicine curriculum for acupuncture students. It was my feeling that an acupuncturist should be able to recognize when to refer a patient for medical support and how to handle emergencies. At the same time, I was teaching a course called "Complementary Healing Systems" at Tufts University School of Medicine, exposing medical students to acupuncture and other nontraditional modalities. A boom in alternative medicine was occurring, and acupuncture was part of it. In 1993, Harvard Medical School's Dr. David Eisenberg published a landmark study quantifying the numbers of people seeking alternatives.

In 1997, however, acupuncture received its biggest boost. The National Institutes of Health (NIH) held a Scientific Consensus Conference to study acupuncture and recommend acupuncture as a treatment for a variety of common conditions. More important, the NIH appeared to approve of the practice of acupuncture in a general way, lending modern medical respect and support to this ancient, metaphysical as well as physical, philosophy. More and more mainstream physicians began to consider acupuncture to be a viable alternative for their patients. Currently, the United Sates has forty acupuncture schools, most offering master's degree programs in acupuncture. Several schools are in the process of developing doctoral curricula, and there is some movement within the acupuncture community to create specialty training. Medical acupuncture has also become more established since the NIH Scientific Consensus Conference Report. In 2000, the AAMA, which surpassed one thousand members, created a board certification for medical acupuncture.

Recently, I have seen my practice change. My colleagues in medicine, who previously might have looked the other way if their patients suggested going to an acupuncturist, now hand out my card or call me, appreciative of having a safe alternative for some of the chronic conditions that they treat. And I have continued to see Chinese medicine in general and the Five-Element system in particular as a lens through which to view my patients, their illnesses, and the road that leads to their health.

Looking back, I am very grateful to have discovered this remarkable healing system. It's enriched my medical practice, and I've spent many gratifying years teaching what I have learned to others. In the following pages, I hope to share with you some of the unique insights that my training in Chinese medicine has given me. You'll learn what acupuncture is, how it works, and what scientific research supports its use. You'll read about the five elements and how they relate to personality and to disease. You'll find a review of the important clinical studies involving acupuncture treatment. And you'll be exposed to the way acupuncture can bridge the gap you may feel between the natural world around you and the health you strive for inside.

# THE UNDERPINNINGS OF ACUPUNCTURE

To MANY AMERICANS, THE NOTION of acupuncture is unfamiliar and foreign. For some, that "strangeness" makes the exploration of acupuncture's history and the use of its techniques to balance and rebalance the body even more exciting. For others, its foreignness becomes a stumbling block that books such as this one hope to clear away.

What's most alien to many Western audiences is the holistic nature of traditional Chinese medicine and its deep ties to the natural world. Health in our culture is individualistic, tied only to the internal workings of our own individual bodies. Even within the body, we narrow the scope of symptoms and disease to separate systems, classifying them according to the organ they most affect—for instance, heart disease or headache—rather than seeing the interconnected nature of the human body and its processes, as practitioners and philosophers do in the East. Furthermore, we in the West have long divided body and mind, failing to recognize how intertwined—if not completely integrated—our physical, psychological, and spiritual natures truly are.

Slowly but steadily, these attitudes are changing as we grow as a culture and as Western medical science recognizes the very real physiological links between and among internal organs, emotional and spiritual influences, and environmental stressors. This chapter introduces you to some of the basic concepts of traditional Chinese medicine so that you too can appreciate the remarkable philosophical underpinnings of this ancient tradition and modern treatment option.

More than twenty-five hundred years ago, a group of healers in China compiled a text known as *The Yellow Emperor's Classic of Internal Medicine*. This treatise on Chinese medicine outlines an approach to life and health still practiced by more than one-quarter of the world's population and increasingly followed here in the United States. In it, we learn that, at its heart, the Chinese philosophy of health is based on the view that humanity, and each individual human, is part of a larger creation—the universe itself. Each of us is subject to the same laws that govern all of nature, including the stars, planets, animals, trees, oceans, and soil. In fact, Chinese medicine refers to the flows of bodily fluid and energy as channels and rivers and to the state of the body as a whole in terms of the natural elements—dryness, heat, cold, dampness, and wind.

According to Chinese philosophy, human beings represent the juncture between heaven and earth and thus are a fusion of cosmic and earthly forces. Indeed, human beings *are* nature and thus are subject to its cyclic pattern and ebbs and flows, and the health of our universe, our planet, our individual bodies, is connected through the same unified system. When any part of this unified whole becomes unbalanced, natural disasters (such as floods or droughts) or human disease may occur. What injures the earth injures each of us, and to heal the body is to foster the health and well-being of the whole universe.

In acupuncture and other Asian healing arts, five major concepts arise out of this philosophy. The first concept, *qi* (pronounced "chee"), a life force of energy, forms the foundation on which two other important ideas are built: *yin-yang* and the five elements. Internal and external causes of disease—the fourth concept—represent environmental, emotional, and lifestyle conditions that affect health and healing. In the fifth concept, the *qi* circulates within the body through twelve primary channels and various secondary channels, which are pathways that bring energy to every cell and organ. These intertwined concepts help to organize and identify physical, emotional, and spiritual information, and to form a guide for practitioners in diagnosing and treating illness.

# *Qi:* The Life Force

According to traditional Asian thought, health is maintained when energy, known as *qi*, is allowed to flow unimpeded throughout the body. *Qi* has been variously translated as "vital force," "vital energy," "spirits," and "breath." Within Asian cultures, *qi* describes the essence of what something is, and the qualities and relationships that define it. *Qi gong* (which means "energy exercise" or "breath exercise") and *tai chi* ("great energy") are movement systems designed to build one's *qi* and move it around the body.

In humans, *qi* is the energy essential for life. In fact, *qi* is synonymous with life itself. It is your *qi* that gives you the energy to walk, talk, think, dream, hope, and love. All the functions of your body and mind are manifestations of *qi*, and the health of your body is determined by a sufficient, balanced, and uninterrupted flow of *qi*. *Qi* ensures bodily functions by keeping blood and other fluids circulating to warm the body, fight disease, and protect the body against negative forces from the external environment.

Chances are you have witnessed *qi* in action and not realized it. For instance, the young athletes on the soccer fields whose kicks, running ability, and competitiveness make them stand out have strong *qi*. People who look as if they have "given up" or as if every step they take is painful have tired *qi*, while those whom we describe as "go-getters" have strong *qi*. In my own life, there are times my wife looks tired or otherwise "off" in the morning. Her blood pressure, weight, blood count, and any other measurements are normal, but I'm seeing something about her vitality or life force. I'm seeing her *qi*.

To understand *qi*, the idea of constant movement and ever repeating cycles and patterns is essential. In fact, the Chinese character for *qi* (the Chinese language is written in a series of pictorial characters that give meaning to the words) is a pot of rice that is boiling, with the steam moving upward. *Qi* involves the activity of life, of metabolism, and of the processing and transformation that turns food into energy.

In Chinese medicine, our *qi* comes from a combination of genetics and lifestyle. It starts with what we bring into the world (called "original *qi*"), which then combines with the *qi* we breathe in as air plus the *qi* in the food we eat. This combination is processed in our organs and becomes the *qi* that flows through the channels. These channels, usually called meridians, are a continuous circuit of pathways throughout the body through which the *qi* circulates. These meridians flow along the surface of the body and through the internal organs, just as underground rivers nourish and support the earth. Located along the meridians are a series of passageways through which you can access and strengthen *qi*, break through blockages, and redirect energy. These acupuncture points can be likened to gates that skilled practitioners can open or shut to influence the direction and flow of energy in the body.

When you are healthy, you have an abundance of *qi* flowing smoothly through the meridians and organs, which allows your body to function harmoniously and in balance. If *qi* becomes blocked along one of your meridians, the organ this energy is meant to nourish will not receive enough *qi* to function. By locating where in the body the *qi* is blocked and then releasing it, acupuncturists attempt to restore proper energy flow to the body.

Although Western medicine has never embraced such concepts, increasing numbers of researchers are beginning to apply their own understanding to the idea of *qi* and its relationship to acupuncture and other methods of Chinese healing. Using sophisticated electromagnetic technology, for instance, scientists have been able to map the electric potential of the skin; more than 90 percent of the skin points that have high electrical conductivity correspond to the acupuncture points that were first used in China thousands of years ago and are still used today.

## *Yin-Yang:* Internal Balance

We live in an age in which we are generally separate from nature. We work under electric lights in buildings with controlled climates, frequently without windows. If we didn't have to travel outside, we might have little idea whether it was cold or hot, morning or evening, humid or dry. Now imagine a time before indoor heating and plumbing, before radio and television, before twenty-four-hour access to the Internet, even before electric lights. When it got dark, people went to sleep; when the sun came up, they awoke. They were always aware of nature and, in fact, were a part of nature.

And, when they looked up, they saw something that was hot, light, and dry. It was dynamic, active, and expansive. It was transcendent; it couldn't be grasped, measured, or quantified. It was the sun; it was heaven. The ancient Chinese described this as *yang*. When they looked down, they saw something that was cooling, moist, solid, dark, and immobile. It held and nourished things; it grew things when given heat and light from above. It wasn't transcendent. It was manifest. It could be held, measured, and quantified. It was earth, and the Chinese called it *yin*.

Nature is a constant cycle from *yin* to *yang* and back again, from winter to summer, from night to day, from the sunny side of the mountain to the shady side. Nature likewise can be seen as a series of *yin-yang* cycles as these seasons repeat themselves within us. We experience birth and infancy, up through adulthood, and on through aging and death. We wake and sleep, get hungry and full, and become active and restful in cycles.

Physiologically, Chinese medicine views parts of the body as having either more *yin* or more *yang* qualities. The same is true of all physiological processes. When you breathe in and expand your lungs and chest cavity, you are in the *yang* phase of respiration. When you exhale, you are in the contractile, *yin* phase. When you are active during the day, you are in the *yang* phase; at rest, you are in *yin*. Food is *yin* substance that the activity of *yang* transforms into tissue and energy.

Remarkably, Western physiology is filled with examples of this *yin-yang* equilibrium. The sympathetic nervous system, which prepares us for fight or flight, can be thought of as a *yang* system, and its partner, the parasympathetic nervous system, governs the *yin* activities of rest and digestion. The systolic pumping of the heart is *yang*; the diastolic relaxation is *yin*. Even our hormonal systems are known to have a diurnal (day-night) variation. The *yang* hormones (such as cortisol and the sex hormones) are active in the daytime, and the *yin* hormones that help the body to rest and regenerate (such as melatonin) are active during the night.

In addition to the physiological functions, every organ of the body likewise has either more *yin* or more *yang* qualities. The *yin* organs are the more solid ones—the heart, spleen, lungs, kidneys, and liver; they are also called *zang* organs. The more functional and hollow organs—the small intestine, stomach, large intestine, and bladder—are the *yang* organs, also known as *fu* organs. The *zang-fu* organs work in mutual support and balance to maintain *yin-yang* balance within the organism as a whole.

According to the principle of *yin-yang*, the body is always striving to maintain a normal state through counterbalances—similar to the Western idea of internal homeostasis. This concept states that our physiology is a constant process of adjusting and readjusting so that we are in a state of balance with our environment. For instance, when it's cold outside, our metabolism responds by increasing and heating us up. Our *yin-yang* balance is not a static condition, but a dynamic equilibrium that moves from *yin* to *yang* and back again as our physical, emotional, and environmental conditions change. When *yin-yang* becomes unbalanced, symptoms of disease may occur.

It's important to realize that *yin* and *yang* are relative, not absolute. We cannot have *yang* all the time, nor *yin* all the time. There's no such thing. In the darkest room, we can begin to see as our eyes adjust to the tiny amounts of light. This is the *yang* within the greater *yin*. No matter how active we are, there must always be a period of rest and inactivity. This is the *yin* that must follow *yang*.

With nonstop activity from our media, our businesses, our homes, and our institutions, we are gradually becoming a society with more and more *yang* and little *yin*. We build more than we allow nature to grow. We value activity and acquisitions more than we value balance and spareness. We sleep less, eat on the run, and spend less time appreciating what we have. There is scarcely room for quiet, for stillness, or to become more receptive to the world around us. The *yin* aspects of the earth such as coolness, moisture, and solitude are overwhelmed by a constant march of global warming, growing deserts, and crowded, busy megacities.

According to *yin-yang* theory, this situation creates imbalance and disease within us and within our natural world. And we are seeing the effects of this in our major illnesses, from cancer (which results largely from a wearing out of the immune system) to chronic fatigue to near epidemic levels of depression. These conditions represent situations in which the body says "enough" and shifts us into a *yin* phase, in which frantic schedules and maximum activity become impossible to sustain.

This need for a quiet *yin* phase to balance the *yang* is not unique to Chinese thought. The ancients of Western culture had similar concepts. In the Bible, every seventh day was to be a day of rest and reflection (our Sabbath), and every seventh year, the land was allowed to regrow and replenish. Every fiftieth year was a jubilee year, in which work was not done, slaves were freed, land was returned to its original owners, and things went back to the way they were originally. This was, in the Judeo-Christian tradition, an acknowledgment of the cycles of activity and rest that are necessary for a healthy life and a healthy world.

The theory of *yin-yang* extends as well to an individual person's character and body structure. Someone with a *yang* body is larger, stronger, and more muscular than someone with a *yin* body. A predominantly *yang* person is likely to enjoy being more active and impulsive, and to thrive in more stimulating and complex settings. A predominantly *yin* personality is more likely to feel comfortable in a relatively quiet, calm environment and to have a more limited capacity for interaction and stress.

Many times, people will choose stimulants or other products that help to correct the "imbalance" of their energy. For instance, someone having more of a *yin* physiology, with its coldness, will be drawn to warm foods. Sometimes, these people, who are more likely to be thin and dry in appearance, will smoke cigarettes, the warmth in their lungs providing them something that is missing. Many people who tend toward extra *yang*, on the other hand, thrive on exercise, which moves the body and provides an outlet for the *yang*. Or, they might like the feeling of a cold beer. These are not necessarily good choices, but on some level, each person is reacting to an imbalance of *yang* and *yin* and attempting to make it better.

An acupuncturist, of course, can address these imbalances much more directly. Many times, he or she will choose a method similar to the one the patient might choose—the person with excess *yang* reaching for the cold beer, for example—that is, adding the opposite condition. Thus, dampness is treated by drying and warming, stagnation is treated by movement, heat is treated by cooling, and so forth. As you'll see further in Chapter 3, the effects of acupuncture points are described not as curing a particular disease, but as increasing the flow of *qi* or as removing blockages from one or more of the channels.

# The Five Elements

The third important concept within traditional Chinese medicine is called the Five-Element or Five-Phase theory, which is concerned with structuring the flow of *qi* and the balance of *yin* and *yang*. This system places all natural phenomena into five categories, each of which represents a stage in the annual progress through the seasons. The five categories are wood (spring), fire (summer), earth (late summer), metal (autumn), and water (winter). Linking the seasons of the year, aspects of nature, and the body's organs, the Five-Phase theory reflects the ever-changing and diverse aspects of nature while providing a unified structure to the universe.

The meaning of the five phases is best understood as a creative cycle, with each phase nourishing and promoting the activities of the next. This cycle is called the *sheng* cycle in Chinese medicine. Spring is a time of birth and rebirth and of rapid growth. There is an increase in activity, an expansion, and a warming. The movement in nature is up and out. This phase of nature is symbolized by wood, like a tree sprout shooting up through the ground. Without the right amount of growth, warmth, moisture, and free movement of the springtime, the full bloom of summer is limited. Thus, spring "creates" summer, or, in Five-Phase theory, wood creates fire.

Summer involves the most activity, with continued growth, maturity, full expansion, and maximum heat. Without the full maturity of blooms, there will be no harvest. In Five-Phase theory, the late summer, or harvest season, is separate from summer and autumn, much as early September feels different to us from mid-July and from late October. In the harvest season, there is stillness and a satisfied feeling to nature, roundness and fullness, and not much movement, with the air frequently heavy and still. Earth, the late summer phase, is created by fire, and earth in turn creates metal. Metal, the autumn, has a declining level of natural activity, an increasing level of coolness and dryness, and a paring down of nature to what is essential.

Metal creates water, which symbolizes the winter—cold, quiet, and with a minimal level of activity on the surface. But winter is actually a time of hidden activity as the seeds that make the next year's growth build their reserves and get ready for the burst of early spring. Without these reserves, there will be no burst. Thus, the water phase is considered the beginning of *yang* in Chinese medicine, and it creates the wood.

In addition to the creative cycle, there is a series of relationships known as the control cycle (sometimes called the "destructive" or *k'o* cycle). This cycle describes the conditions whereby one phase limits or controls another. Fire controls metal, since it is the warmth of fire that makes metal malleable. Metal controls wood, as an ax cuts a tree and a gardener's tools define the boundaries of a garden. Wood controls earth, its root systems holding and shaping it. Earth controls water, as the banks of a river create the conduit through which water flows. And water controls fire by its moisture and cooling properties.

Since you are part of nature, these relationships also take place within your body, and the skilled practitioner uses diagnostic information to understand them and how they affect your health. Each phase of the five phases is paired with two organs: one *yin* and one *yang*. Spring/wood is associated with the liver (*yin*) and gallbladder (*yang*); summer/fire with the heart (*yin*) and small intestine (*yang*); late summer/earth with the spleen (*yin*) and stomach (*yang*); autumn/metal with the lungs (*yin*) and large intestine (*yang*); and winter /water with the kidneys (*yin*) and bladder (*yang*). In addition, there are two functions that are not associated with organs but that relate to the summer/fire phase. These are the triple heater (*yang*) and the pericardium (*yin*).

Colors, emotions, senses, and flavors are also related to the five phases and to the human body. By viewing the body in this framework, practitioners diagnose and treat illnesses in a highly personal and individual way.

In Part II, the phases and how they relate to disease and health are explored in more depth; for now, let's take a brief look at each to see how they correspond with physical, emotional, and natural cycles and the health of the body.

## THE FIVE PHASES AND CORRESPONDENCES

|  | WOOD | FIRE | EARTH | METAL | WATER |
|---|---|---|---|---|---|
| *YIN* ORGAN | Liver | Heart/ Pericardium | Spleen | Lungs | Kidneys |
| *YANG* ORGAN | Gallbladder | Small intestine/ Triple heater | Stomach | Large intestine | Bladder |
| SEASON | Spring | Summer | Late summer | Autumn | Winter |
| CLIMATE | Wind | Heat | Dampness | Dryness | Cold |
| NOURISHES | Tendons Ligaments | Blood vessels | Flesh Muscles | Skin Hair | Bones |
| EMOTION | Anger | Joy | Sympathy | Grief | Fear |
| COLOR | Green | Red | Yellow | White | Blue |
| FLAVOR | Sour | Bitter | Sweet | Pungent | Salty |
| ODOR | Rancid | Scorched | Fragrant | Rotten | Putrid |
| SOUND | Shout | Laugh | Sing | Weep | Groan |

## *Wood—Spring/Wind: Liver* (Yin) *and Gallbladder* (Yang)

Wood is the element of spring. Wood energy is focused and strong, always pushing against boundaries to grow, just as plants push up through the soil to grow every springtime. The *zang-fu* organs of the wood phase are the liver and the gallbladder.

Emotionally and spiritually, the liver—which is the *yin* organ of the wood phase and known as the "planner" of the body—governs growth and development, ambitions, and creativity. Obstruction of liver energy can cause intense feelings of frustration, rage, and anger, and in turn, such feelings can cause further disturbance of liver energy and liver function. The *yang* organ of the wood phase is the gallbladder, also known as the "honorable minister" or the "decision maker." The gallbladder governs daring and decisiveness; even in English, having "gall" means having a lot of nerve.

### Fire—Summer/Heat:
### Heart (Yin) and Small Intestine (Yang)

As the heat of its corresponding season of summer suggests, fire has a hot and passionate energy. It represents the spark of life and joy, and people with this energy radiate warmth and thrive on interpersonal contact.

In Chinese as well as Western tradition, the heart—fire's *yin* organ—is thought of as the "king" of the body. It commands the other organs, houses the spirit, and controls the emotions. According to *The Yellow Emperor's Classic*, the heart is "the sovereign of all organs and represents the consciousness of one's being. It is responsible for intelligence, wisdom, and spiritual transformation." The word for heart in Chinese is *hsin*, which means "mind." The heart also houses the *shen*, or spirit. This shows just how integrated spirit, emotion, intellect, and physicality are within the Eastern tradition.

Have you ever noticed that after periods of intense emotional release, you're more likely to catch a cold or suffer from a headache? That's because the heart is also integral to the function of the immune system; when the fire energy and the heart are strong, the immune system protects the body against diseases. When they are weak, the body becomes vulnerable.

The small intestine is fire energy's *yang* organ. Also known as the "minister of sorting," this organ sorts out the pure from the impure in the food you ingest, sending the pure to the spleen, where it is transformed into *qi*, and the impure to the large intestine for elimination. A similar process takes place on the emotional and spiritual levels. If your system imbalance affects the small intestine, you have trouble discriminating between the pure and impure in your relationships, your career, and other aspects of life.

Fire also has two functions associated with it. One, the *yin* function, is the pericardium, also referred to as "circulation-sex" or "heart protector." The pericardium, like the membrane it is named for, acts as the guard to the inner sanctum of the heart, allowing for circulation throughout the body. The *yang* function, the triple heater, distributes heat and energy through the three areas of the body—upper, middle, and lower.

### Earth—Late Summer/Dampness: Spleen (Yin) and Stomach (Yang)

As its name implies, earth energy is rich and nourishing. The earth element—and its corresponding internal organs—concern eating and digestion and nourishing the body, mind, and spirit. When the earth phase is in balance, it forms a serene, stable center of gravity. People with a strong earth energy tend to be well grounded and empathic, able to step into another's shoes—and back into their own—with ease, which is why the earth energy is also known as the mothering energy.

But when that energy is upset, discomfort arises. Emotionally, someone with imbalanced earth energy can feel empty and out of balance and can be overly worried and meddlesome. Physically, an earth-energy dysfunction is fairly easy to identify because it results in nausea, excess gas, and other intestinal disorders involving its *yin-yang* organs.

Called the "minister of transportation," the spleen, earth's *yin* organ, receives food from the small intestine and transforms it into *qi*. It also keeps the blood flowing in its proper channels. Appropriately, the stomach, earth's *yang* organ, is called the "sea of nourishment." It is responsible for providing the entire system with energy from the digestion of food and fluids. A dysfunction of the stomach can thus lead to imbalances in any and all parts of the body.


## Metal—Autumn/Dryness: Lungs (Yin) and Large Intestine (Yang)

The traditional symbol of metal energy is a snowcapped mountain, firmly grounded in the earth but reaching with power toward the heavens. Metal energy is one of striving and of bringing in what the body and soul need (through the lungs) and letting go of the impure (through the large intestine). In emotional terms, the lungs balance the ability to demand (breathing in) and the ability to release (exhaling). When metal energy is out of balance, the body and the soul cannot let go; thinking becomes rigid, and the body begins to stiffen.

The lungs, the *yin* organ of the metal phase, are called the "prime minister" because they control breath and energy as well as assist the heart in circulating the blood. Proper breathing is thus essential to maintain balance and health throughout the body. It also helps to regulate the autonomic nervous system, which is responsible for maintaining a regular pulse and blood pressure.

The *yang* organ of the metal phase is the large intestine, also known as the "minister of elimination." It controls the transformation of digestive wastes from liquid to solid and then transports the waste for excretion. It plays an important role in maintaining the balance and purity of bodily fluids. An imbalance within the *yang* metal phase often results in cramping and constipation.

## Water—Winter/Cold:
## Kidneys (Yin) and Bladder (Yang)

The power of water nourishes the body, mind, and spirit with energy. In fact, water represents a spiritual and directed type of energy, and water types tend to be introspective as well as fascinated with the pursuit of knowledge. Water is also a sexual energy; although the heart is the center of emotional passion and intimacy, the kidneys (the *yin* water organ) hold the key to physical sexual potency and performance.

Known as the "minister of power," the kidneys are regarded as the body's most important reservoir of essential energy. They are also responsible for creating and dispersing warmth and energy throughout the body. The kidneys also store *jing*, our genetic reserves. *Jing* represents the reserve of energy each of us has that buffers us from life's steady wear and tear. Those with lots of *jing* in reserve stay healthier and are more energetic than those without it. Having *jing* gives us our sexual energy, our ability to withstand stresses without a breakdown in our bodies, and the chance for longevity.

The bladder is called the "minister of reserve" because it stores and then excretes the urinary waste fluids that are passed down from the kidneys. The bladder and the kidneys also are both intimately related to the autonomic nervous system and thus react to stress; inflammation of all kinds—redness of the eyes, muscle soreness—as well as exhaustion and lethargy may result.

Emotionally, a person with an imbalance of water energy may become fixed and stubborn instead of exhibiting the free-flowing direction that is his or her usual nature. Panic may result, and many people with an imbalance of water energy suffer with panic disorder and chronic fatigue syndrome. (Common symptoms of chronic fatigue syndrome include substantial impairment in short-term memory or concentration, sore throat, tender lymph nodes, muscle pain, and pain in multiple joints [without swelling or redness].)

# The Internal and External Causes of Disease

Centuries ago, practitioners of Chinese medicine observed that climatic conditions—heat, cold, dampness, and so on—affected the health of their patients. These practitioners also accepted that strong, untempered emotions can influence internal physiological changes. These external and internal factors continue to be used as tools to diagnose and treat disease.

## *The External Causes of Disease*

The six external causes of disease include the five climates, which are wind, heat, dampness, dryness, and cold; whenever one of the climates dominates within any part of the body, illness and imbalance result. The sixth external condition, extreme heat—or fire—derives from an extreme external environmental situation.

*Wind*  The nature of wind is unpredictable movement that disturbs the natural location and direction of all things, including the *qi* that flows within the channels. Wind is associated with the wood element and the spring season. However, wind occurs in all seasons and thus takes on the prevailing climatic conditions associated with each season. In summer, for instance, there may be a heat wind; in winter, a cold wind is possible. The unpredictability of wind makes it a frequent cause of disease, particularly when it's combined with other climatic causes. Sometimes, excess energy can accumulate within an organ and suddenly move to another organ according to the control or creative cycles of the five phases. The resulting wind condition can either overstimulate an organ or suppress its energy.

A prime example of a wind condition is tic douloureux, also known as trigeminal neuralgia, a painful condition that comes on suddenly (often after the person is exposed to a draft) and severely. Wind illness—in this case, a cold damp wind—may also be exemplified by some cases of fibromyalgia, in which the pain moves around the body, frequently being relieved by heat and movement.

*Heat* Heat is the prevailing energy of summer and corresponds with the fire phase. As is true for wind, heat may also occur in other seasons, taking on their prevailing conditions, so that you may have a damp heat in late summer or a dry heat in autumn. Excess heat causes headaches, chronic thirst, and excessive sweating; it can also overstimulate any of the organs or organ networks. Hyperthyroidism, with its heat and sweating, tremors, and overactivity, is a classic heat condition.

*Dampness* Dampness is related to the late summer and corresponds with the earth phase. Its essential quality is that of humidity, which seeps through the body, leading to fatigue, lethargy, bloating, and cold sweats. In the body, dampness is the result of something's not being processed, including both food and thoughts. When dampness accumulates, it can turn to phlegm, which is denser and more likely to cause stagnation and imbalance. Dampness may suppress organ function. It can also occur in combination with other energies to produce such conditions as cold dampness and wind dampness. A patient who has swollen, heavy ankles has a "cold dampness" condition, while someone with an arthritic swelling of the joints has damp heat in those joints.

*Dryness* Related to autumn and corresponding with the metal phase, external dryness is caused by insufficient moisture in the air and is particularly damaging to the lungs. Internal dryness usually implies a deficiency of *yin*, with its loss of moistening and cooling. When combined with other energies, dryness can cause a host of symptoms, including hot spells (heat dryness) and chronic dry cough (cold dryness). Menopause is a situation in which menstrual bleeding has ceased and the body's moisture has decreased, leading to dryness. In former times, before indoor heating kept houses warm, cold dryness was a frequent external cause of disease.

*Cold* The cold climate is associated with the water element and—as its name implies—the winter season. When cold invades the system from the external environment, it causes chills, fever, and headache. If cold settles in the abdominal organs, diarrhea, gas, and cramping may result. Internal cold, on the other hand, arises from having deficient *yang* in the vital organs. Someone with this condition may suffer from chilled hands and feet as well as sexual impotence.

*Fire* Chinese medicine distinguishes the sudden, overwhelming exposure to extreme heat from the lesser, more chronic problem of heat. Such an external cause of disease is sometimes called "extreme heat" so as not to confuse it with the element fire. Examples of this type of exposure are sunstroke and heatstroke, as well as actually being in a building that is on fire.


## The Internal Causes of Disease

Although Western medicine has resisted the idea that emotions can directly affect physical health, evidence to confirm the connection has emerged in recent decades. Perhaps the most striking example is the acceptance of the type A personality—denoting someone who reacts to his or her environment with tension, impatience, ambition, and perfectionism—and its relationship to an increased risk of heart disease. Eastern medicine has long recognized this connection and continues to use the emotional condition of a patient as a factor in diagnosis and treatment.

*Anger* In this context, anger isn't usually the explosive burst of rage you experience when you're cut off in traffic, but rather the constant dissatisfaction, resentment, and frustration that tightens the muscles and makes you chronically unhappy. When it does not move, it becomes stuck, resulting in stagnation, particularly in the wood channels.

*Joy* Appropriate joy and happiness are, of course, beneficial to health. However, some people are "over the top," laughing at everything, with no real control. This type of inappropriate joy is considered damaging to the heart and can burn out the fire energy, leading to flatness and depression.

*Excess Cogitation* Part of the earth energy depends on movement and processing, and when thoughts become obsessive and never go anywhere, they can accumulate into dampness and phlegm.

*Worry* A form of excess cogitation, worry is tinged more with fear. Excess worry and anxiety will eventually paralyze the energy, obstructing new movement and growth.

*Grief* Here again, appropriate grief is healthy. However, when grieving extends for months or years without resolution, or when everything seems to represent a source of loss, the metal organs of grieving, the lungs and large intestine, are affected, usually with a dryness that leads to weakness of the *qi*.

*Fear* The water element is deep seated, and fear can paralyze you deeply, imparting a sense that nothing is safe. This does not have to be fear of anything specific, but just an overwhelming sense of fear or panic. The effect is less energy in the kidneys and bladder, which leads to fatigue and low reserves.

*Fright* Acute fright is seen as a separate internal cause of disease. An example is experiencing something horrible and being unable to let go of the experience and therefore unable to proceed with one's life.

# The Twelve Primary Channels and Secondary Channels

The final concept necessary to understanding the fundamentals of traditional Chinese healing is the channels. As noted earlier, *qi* moves in cycles timed by natural phenomena, and it circulates within the human body through what is called the *jing-luo* network of channels. On these channels lie the *xue*, or holes, to which this book refers as acupoints.

There are many ways of classifying the channels, and the different systems of acupuncture group the channels differently, although the points and channel locations are similar. The most common way of naming channels is for the organ with which they are associated, since each channel sends a deep branch of *qi* flow into a solid *yin* (*zang*) or hollow *yang* (*fu*) organ. Thus, the channels are called heart, small intestine, bladder, kidney, and so forth.

Another way of classifying channels is used primarily in the French energetics system of acupuncture, popular among U.S. physician acupuncturists. It divides the channels into Six Greater Divisions, according to where in the cycle of *yin* and *yang* they are active. Each of these divisions is further divided into its upper and lower portions (frequently named for the organ with which it is associated). Thus, the *tai yang* (greater *yang*) channel is made up of the upper *tai yang* (small intestine, on the arm) and lower *tai yang* (bladder, on the leg).

When contemplating the use of the channels to treat a patient, an acupuncturist generally considers the areas of the body that the channels traverse, their *yin-yang* characteristics, and the functions of the organs to which each channel homes.

An example is a patient with back pain. By taking a careful medical history, the acupuncturist learns that the person urinates frequently and

## SUMMARY OF THE TWELVE PRIMARY CHANNELS

| 12 MERIDIANS | 6 GREATER MERIDIANS | LOCATION |
| --- | --- | --- |
| Heart | Upper *shao yin* (lesser *yin*) | Inside front of arm |
| Small intestine | Upper *tai yang* (greater *yang*) | Inside back of arm |
| Bladder | Lower *tai yang* | Outside back of leg |
| Kidney | Lower *shao yin* | Inside front of leg |
| Pericardium | Upper *jue yin* (limit of *yin*) | Middle front of arm |
| Triple heater | Upper *shao yang* (lesser *yang*) | Middle back of arm |
| Gallbladder | Lower *shao yang* | Middle back of leg |
| Liver | Lower *jue yin* | Middle front of leg |
| Lung | Upper *tai yin* (greater *yin*) | Outside front of arm |
| Large intestine | Upper *yang ming* (sunlight *yang*) | Inside back of arm |
| Stomach | Lower *yang ming* | Inside back of leg (actually on the front) |
| Spleen | Lower *tai yin* | Outside front of leg |

is cold intolerant; that is, warmth feels good to the patient, particularly on the back. These symptoms tell the acupuncturist that the problem lies within the tai *yang*, or bladder channel, which goes longitudinally up the back. The tai *yang* is a water channel and so tends toward cold, and it involves what the body reserves, including the holding capacity of the bladder organ. The treatment will typically involve heating the channel as well as using needles.

Following is a description of the twelve primary channels and where they exist in the body.

*The Heart Channel* Starting inside the chest at the heart, the heart channel surfaces in the armpit and runs downward through the inner surface of the upper arm, elbow, forearm, and wrist, to end near the fifth fingernail. A branch runs inside the chest to the small intestine.

*The Small Intestine Channel* This channel starts on the fifth fingernail and runs up the outer surface of the wrist, forearm, elbow, upper arm, and back of the shoulder to the back of the neck. It then passes through the jaw hinge, to end in front of the ear. At the shoulder, a branch runs inside the body to the heart and the small intestine.

*The Bladder Channel* The bladder channel starts at the upper inner corner of the eye and runs upward over the top of the head and down the back of the head and neck. It flows down the back in two streams to the buttocks, down the back of the thigh, knee, and calf to the outer ankle, and ends at the fifth toenail. A branch runs from the back inside to the bladder and kidneys.

*The Kidney Channel* This channel underneath the foot runs from the instep to the inner ankle. It travels up the inner surface of the calf to the knee and thigh until it reaches the abdomen near the middle of the body. From there, it goes up the abdomen to the chest, along the breast-bone, ending just below the clavicle on the edge of the sternum. On the abdomen, a branch runs inside to the kidneys and bladder and also connects to the heart.

*The Pericardium Channel* This channel starts inside the chest at the tissue that surrounds the heart (called the pericardium). It then surfaces just lateral to the breast and runs over the shoulder and down through the inner surface of the upper arm, elbow, forearm, and wrist, to end on the middle fingernail. A branch runs from inside the chest to the triple heater, another channel.

*The Triple Heater Channel* This channel starts on the fourth finger-nail and runs over the back of the hand to the wrist, forearm, elbow, and upper arm, to the back of the shoulder, and then across the shoulder to the side of the neck. It ends at the outside of the eyebrow. A branch leaves the main channel at the shoulder and runs inside the body, where it connects to the three body cavities that give the channel its name.

*The Gallbladder Channel* This channel starts at the temple and travels around the top of the ear and then forward to above the eyebrow. It then goes back across the head to the back of the neck and down the side of the ribs. It then goes around the hip joint and behind it, and travels down the side of the upper and lower leg and across the ankle to the foot, ending by the fourth toenail. One internal channel travels from the gallbladder channel on the leg to the liver channel, and another leaves the channel in the torso, traveling to the gallbladder organ.

*The Liver Channel* This channel starts by the big toenail and runs up the top of the foot to the ankle, up the shin to the knee, and inside the thigh to the groin. It then circles the genitals, ascends the abdomen, and ends at the lower border of the ribs. A branch leaves the main channel at the abdomen and runs inside to the stomach, liver, and gallbladder, and up through the lungs to the back of the nose and the crown of the head.

*The Lung Channel* The lung channel starts in the lungs, inside the chest, and surfaces in front of the shoulder. It runs through the shoulder and down the inner surface of the upper arm, elbow, forearm, and wrist, to end next to the thumbnail. A branch runs from inside the chest to the large intestine.

*The Large Intestine Channel* This channel starts at the index finger-nail and runs up through the wrist, forearm, upper arm, and shoulder, up the side of the neck in the belly of the sternomastoid muscle, and around the mouth, to its end at the side of the nose. A branch leaves the main channel at the shoulder and runs inside the body to the lungs and large intestine.

*The Stomach Channel* Starting just below the eye, this channel runs down the face to the corner of the mouth, through the jaw upward to the temple, and down the front of the neck to the center of the breast. From there, it flows to the abdomen and then to the outer thigh, knee, shin, and ankle, ending by the second toenail. From the clavicle, a branch of the stomach channel runs to the stomach and spleen.

*The Spleen Channel* This channel starts by the big toe, runs up the instep to the ankle, and moves up the inside portion of the shin to the knee, thigh, and groin. It continues on up the abdomen and chest, to end below the armpit. From the abdomen, a branch runs inside the body to the spleen, connecting to the stomach and joining the heart.

In addition to the Twelve Primary Channels, other groupings of channels have significance in acupuncture theory and treatment. For instance, there are tendinomuscular channels, which are superficial channels that give *qi* to the tendons and muscles through which they pass. There are deep channels called Distinct Meridians that bring energy directly to the *zang-fu* organs. But the most widely used are probably the Eight Extraordinary Meridians, thus called because they act as great reservoirs of energy for the other channels. Of the eight, only the following two actually have separate points on the body; the others are made up of points on the primary channels.

### The Ren *Channel (Also Known as Conception Vessel)*

This channel holds the *yin* energy of the body and covers the *yin*, or front, surface of the body. Here, it acts like the ocean, feeding and receiving *qi* from the twelve channels. It starts in front of the anus just below the genitals and runs upward along the midline to the abdomen, through the navel, and up the chest to the neck. It continues in the midline over the chin, to end just below the lower lip.

### The Du *Channel (Also Known as Governing Vessel)*

This channel is the reservoir for the *yang* energy of the body and thus traverses the *yang*, or back, surface. It begins at the tip of the coccyx just above the anus and follows the spine upward to the back of the neck, over the midline of the skull. It descends down the nose, to end in the middle of the upper lip.

Together, these two channels hold the body's *yin* and *yang* energy, which cycle in and out in a microcirculation. Several systems of Chinese meditation and *qi gong* involve concentrating on the circulation through the Governing and Conception Vessels. Along all of these channels runs *qi*, the essence of life, the primal energy. If the pathways are open and free flowing, *qi* will nourish and energize the organs and substances throughout. However, if a blockage exists, imbalance results, with more *qi* running to certain organs, which depletes other organs of the energy they need to thrive. Acupuncture—the exacting use of needles to manipulate the energy as it flows—works to restore the proper flow of *qi* and thus balance and health to the body.

If you're like most people new to the theories and principles of traditional Chinese medicine in general, or acupuncture in particular, no doubt you're asking yourself, "But *how* does acupuncture work to heal my body and mind?" As you'll see in the next chapter, Western science is now trying to answer that question in language and concepts more familiar to Western sensibilities. However, it's important to realize—and this caveat is stressed throughout the book—that the beauty and the power of traditional Chinese medicine may simply not translate into the definitions of medicine developed in the West.

3

# HOW ACUPUNCTURE WORKS
## The Theories

THE CONCEPT OF USING ENERGY channels to explain health and ill-ness—to say nothing of classifying physiological and intellectual functions in terms of seasons and climates—sounds mystical and even irrational to many Westerners, particularly physicians. Nevertheless, because acupuncture and other forms of traditional Chinese healing have been successful for thousands of years, scientists in the West have in recent decades attempted to explain how acupuncture works from their own perspective. Fortunately or unfortunately, these efforts will ultimately fail, because traditional Chinese medicine is based on concepts and perhaps even physical manifestations that simply cannot be translated into the Western lexicon.

The goal, however, is a worthy one: an understanding of acupuncture from the perspective of Western medical science would help build a bridge to mainstream medicine and increase its acceptance. And the results so far have been encouraging, with several theories correlating well with the idea of energy pathways running through the body, as is theorized in traditional Chinese medicine. Before exploring these theories, it's important to understand some of the built-in limitations of such a discussion.

## Proving a Western Basis: The Challenges

It's hard to cite two more different ways of looking at the human body—and the world—than the Eastern and Western philosophies. The central issue within traditional Chinese medicine is not how acupuncture and other forms of treatment work; what mechanism is actually responsible for returning balance and health to a particular individual is almost beside the point. Instead, both historically and practically, the practitioner focuses on when and in what way to use the treatment options available.

To be fair to the Western medical establishment, understanding even the fundamentals—never mind the intricacies—of Chinese medicine is a daunting task, requiring intensive research into centuries of philosophy, history, and economics, to say nothing of unfamiliar medical techniques and approaches. Because of this, past attempts at translating and assimilating traditional Chinese medical concepts and paradigms have not always been successful, resulting in a host of texts with inaccurate descriptions of theories and practices. Thus, when current researchers attempt to first understand and then "prove" the dynamics of this complicated science, they begin with several false premises that lead, necessarily, to false conclusions.

Fortunately, as Stephen J. Birch and Robert L. Felt recount in their book *Understanding Acupuncture* (Churchill Livingstone, 1999), several scholars and researchers are taking a new look into the misappropriations and mistranslations of the past. Others are attempting to bridge the gap by explaining the effects of treatment, particularly acupuncture treatment, on the body in well-understood, Western, biomedical terms. A few of those theories are described later in this chapter.

Despite the strides, challenges remain. Several entrenched Western medical concepts interfere—perhaps fatally—with the goal of completely assimilating traditional Chinese medicine into our own culture. Among those obstacles are the following Western concepts:

• *Division of mind, body, and spirit* As discussed in Chapter 2, the Eastern philosophy of health includes consciousness (intellect) and spirit as integral parts of the medical dynamic. However, the intellect and the spirit have no physical correlates here in the West, and thus, they are impossible to measure or assess by Western medical standards. In the East, doctors do not recognize a distinction between psychological and physical illnesses, neither in their diagnoses nor in their treatments. An emotional upset contributes directly to the balance of the entire system and may even affect certain organ networks more than others. Granted, the concept that stress—loosely defined as emotional pressure from the external environment—has debilitating effects on health has gained some ground among mainstream Western physicians, but that's about as close as we've come to accepting the idea that a person's brains, emotions, and body are one and the same thing.

• *View of disease as isolated and discrete* Western medicine focuses on individual organs rather than on interconnections; our ideas about health and disease stem from the level of specific and discrete organ systems, organs, tissues, and cells. In the East, the view is holistic, marked by a unified emphasis on the entire body, mind, and spirit as an integrated entity. While the Western tradition locates the cause of a disorder in a single organ or system, in the East, a problem in one organ may stem from an imbalance in any of a number of areas and in turn cause further dysfunction throughout the body. Because of this fundamental difference in approach, East and West cannot even agree on the name of disorders. The word *asthma*, for instance, has no meaning in the East, where a practitioner would call the breathing problems and allergic response "kidney not grasping the *qi* of the lung," "damp heat accumulation," or "wind invading the lung," depending on the patient's unique constitutional makeup and symptoms.

Treatment is equally dissimilar, in both purpose and methodology. In the West, we target treatments to the specific organ or system we deem "diseased." To carry forward the asthma example, we develop and prescribe drugs that attack the collapsing bronchial tubes or tamper down the allergic response. In the East, the course of treatment depends entirely on where the practitioner locates the root source of the imbalance in that patient's body. The lungs may not be treated at all in addressing asthmatic symptoms, if the cause is elsewhere. Furthermore, because traditional Chinese medicine is by nature "inexact" and highly subjective, two practitioners may diagnose the same patient in markedly different ways, depending on their training, their philosophies, and their techniques.

• *Requirement of objective criteria to assess accuracy of diagnosis and effectiveness of treatment*  The challenges in understanding and accepting even the most basic definitions of health and disease are only part of the problem. Even if it were possible to do so on a personal or institutional level, evaluating Chinese medicine is still a major hurdle because of the standards to which we hold medical "facts." In Western medicine, the randomized controlled trial is the gold standard of medical investigation. This method involves randomly dividing one large set of patients into two or more treatment groups without telling them to which group they belong. One group, called the control group, receives a placebo (inactive) treatment while the other group receives the "real" treatment.

This approach features at least two problems and one essential fallacy, when it is used to evaluate the efficacy of acupuncture. The first problem, as discussed previously, is that it is difficult, if not impossible, to standardize either the diagnosis or the treatment among a large group of people, even those with similar symptoms. The approach is in fact anathema to traditional Chinese medicine. Second, even in trials that extend over several months, many Chinese practitioners contend that the timing is too limited, maintaining that the effects of acupuncture are much subtler and develop much more slowly than Western treatments. In support of this argument, evidence exists that acupuncture effects may continue to emerge long after the practitioner finishes the patient's course of treatment.

The essential fallacy about randomized controlled trials is the premise that a "placebo effect," which is what the control group experiences, is any less real or important than the active treatment. *Placebo* is Latin for "I shall please," and Western medical science has generally defined it as a soothing but ineffective result. However, as researcher Stephen Birch points out, the placebo effect involves specific physiological mechanisms, including the release of endorphins, body chemicals that act to relieve pain. These mechanisms are probably triggered by factors that Western science has difficulty evaluating or accepting, including the influence that a caring physician has on a patient and how much a patient believes in the treatment and wants to get well.

It's possible that scientists could create an ideal placebo, one that would trigger a predictable and appropriate response in most patients who take it. In one study, the color of the placebo pill made a significant difference on whether the patient considered it to be effective. Also, several studies have documented that the way in which questions are asked during a medical exam (i.e., sympathetically, or cold and clinically) can alter the patient's impression of whether the visit was helpful or not. And studies show that if the patient believes a treatment will work, the results will be better, whether the treatment is a placebo or not.

With acupuncture, the difficulty of using randomized controlled trials is compounded by the method of treatment itself. Acupuncture is, first and foremost, a system that uses needles for its effects. It's extremely difficult to convince people that they've been needled if they have not been. So, studies that compare needling with no needling are flawed, and instead, researchers have used something called "sham acupuncture," in which points that are not on acupuncture diagrams and are therefore thought to be inactive are needled as placebos.

Acupuncture gets even more mysterious as we take a closer look at channels and points. As explained later in the chapter, we may not be talking about discrete channels that are visible, such as arteries or nerves. We may be talking instead about energy fields that have certain direction, signaling points, and spatial orientation. So, if we stick a point that's not a known acupuncture point and therefore supposedly sham, it may still have some effect on the energy.

As a consequence, we get a result such as that from one study of acupuncture's effectiveness in treating back pain. Here, acupuncture was deemed better than no acupuncture for the treatment of back pain, but sham acupuncture and real acupuncture were equally effective! Recently, there have been novel attempts to get around this needle problem. For instance, researchers are testing a device that will shield the view of the needle from the patient, and either a real needle or a skin sensation that feels like a needle prick will be given. It remains to be seen whether these new devices will open new avenues of acupuncture research. Also, in what are known as crossover studies, half of the patients are treated with acupuncture, and half are not; after a measured amount of time, the groups are switched and the results compared. Presumably, when a group has acupuncture, the members will show greater effects.

A debate proceeds within the alternative-medicine community in general regarding whether the randomized controlled format is the best way of studying these types of healing systems. Developed to research single drugs and their specific effects, randomized controlled studies may not be the best way of investigating complex healing systems and their treatments. Some alternative-medicine researchers—including Lukoff, Edwards, and Miller in a 1998 article in *Alternative Therapy*—suggest using a type of research that includes the accumulation of single case studies, which, when performed carefully and scientifically, yields accurate and valuable information.

One way of avoiding the natural bias involved in studying acupuncture to treat "asthma" is to study the Chinese medicine diagnoses. That is, rather than study acupoints X and Y to treat asthma, we might ask several experienced acupuncturists to evaluate the asthma patients. Only patients who have the same syndrome—for instance, "wind heat invading the lung"—would be included in the study, and the treatment would be standardized.

The need for such an approach raises the last major issue regarding the clinical study of acupuncture. A minimum number (called *n*) of cases is necessary to have a statistically significant result. Since acupuncture is just hitting the mainstream, we haven't reached *n* with the number of people treated for any one condition. Therefore, many researchers believe we do not have enough information to provide a clear result. Thus, the bulk of acupuncture clinical studies, many of which show promising results, have methodological flaws that make the effectiveness of acupuncture subject to ongoing debate.

The good news is that, despite the obstacles, the medical establishment appears willing and able to continue its investigation into acupuncture's efficacy, and along many avenues.

# The Physiology of Acupuncture

A practitioner of acupuncture makes a diagnosis by touching and smelling the patient's skin, measuring twelve pulses along both arms, and examining the tongue. The practitioner then punctures the skin at specific points with needles, sometimes heating the needles or the acupoints by placing a burning herb called *moxa* on or near them, and waits. When asked to explain the process, the practitioner describes a pattern of energy that flows through the body, through nature, through the universe, an energy that the practitioner hopes to redirect, using the needles to bring the body back into a state of balance and health.

To a medical doctor trained in the Western paradigm of medicine, this approach to diagnosis and treatment—and health and disease—seems completely foreign. To one who understands the human body as a set of organs and processes, such an approach seems mysterious and—if one is closed to all but the most empirical evidence evaluated by Western standards—absolutely improbable. How could needles placed on particular points on the body affect internal organs and physiological processes?

As noted earlier, that question, which continues to intrigue scientists throughout the Western world, may be inappropriate, or at least unnecessary. Furthermore, any answers to it that scientists develop may never be settled, because the answers cannot be translated into a set of facts that we in the West know how to interpret.

Nevertheless, we continue our attempts to explain acupuncture's effects on the body in terms acceptable and rational to a Western scientific perspective. These attempts began in the early 1970s, prompted by the publication of reporter James Reston's articles about his experience with acupuncture as an analgesic after his surgery in China. For many years, the investigation into the mechanisms involved in acupuncture pertained almost solely to its pain-relieving, pain-blocking effects. Although this research yielded some relevant and valid results, it represented a skewed approach to the science of acupuncture until recent years. During the past decade or so, especially, investigations into other mechanisms that might explain acupuncture's efficacy have pointed in interesting directions, some of which are discussed in this section. So far, however, scientists have not found any direct relationship between acupuncture points and specific anatomical structures. For instance, acupuncture channels do not follow nerve root patterns, and acupoints do not reliably correspond to muscles or tendons. Nor has any researcher been able to define *qi* as a physiological entity or process that we would understand from a Western perspective.

On the other hand, studies do indicate that acupuncture points are physiologically unique areas of the body. Specifically, the areas around the acupoints tend to have a higher concentration of peripheral nerves and a higher electrical conductivity than tissue in other areas of the body. Moreover, many measurable biological changes, including increases in blood pressure and white blood cell counts, occur during and following treatment with acupuncture. Therefore, without question, acupuncture works not just as a placebo, as discussed in the previous section, but also in as yet undefined ways to help restore health and balance in the body. Among the lines of research are the following theories, some of which are quite promising.

## The Placebo Theory

Some researchers believe that at least part of the reason that acupuncture works is that patients *want* the treatment to alleviate their condition or *believe* that it will alleviate it, or both. This explanation is controversial for several reasons. First of all, stimulation of acupuncture points produces a wide variety of physiological responses, including changes in blood pressure, temperature, and blood cell count. These changes themselves are certainly responsible for some of the healing effects of acupuncture.

Second, as mentioned earlier, a debate still rages over the types of placebo studies performed and their methodology. The research is not accepted by some authorities and, in certain cases, may produce inaccurate results. The fact is, at least in regard to treating pain, many studies show that acupuncture works about 70 to 80 percent of the time, compared with only 30 percent for placebo treatments.

## The Neurological Theory

In 1975, two researchers, Melzak and Wall, articulated the Gate Control theory of nerve transmission. The premise is that acupuncture primarily affects the nervous system, causing it to block the pain stimuli and, at the same time, produce pain-relieving messages. According to this theory, acupuncture activates small nerve fibers in the muscle, which send impulses to the spinal cord. The spinal cord, midbrain, and hypothalamus-pituitary axis receive the messages and then both block pain signals and dull the pain signals that get through.

Because more peripheral nerves are located near acupoints and because these areas have greater electric conductivity, this theory appears to have merit. However, it falls short of explaining several aspects of acupuncture. For one, acupuncture has been shown to effectively treat a wide variety of conditions apart from pain. For another, acupuncture's effects continue long after needling ceases; if it worked only when the nerves were being stimulated, the pain and other symptoms would return as soon as the practitioner removed the needles.

## The Neurohumoral Theory

Far more persuasive and inclusive is the neurohumoral theory, first developed in the 1970s after scientists discovered the body chemicals called endorphins. Endorphins act to inhibit pain transmission by triggering pleasure centers in the brain and other nervous tissue. In one study, Dr. Bruce Pomeranz measured an increase in endorphin levels after stimulating patients' acupuncture points on the ears. He later determined that acupuncture stimulates what are called "type 3 small afferent fibers" within the muscle tissue. These fibers are connected to the hypothalamus-pituitary axis, which is an important link in the nervous system's response to pain. The hypothalamus-pituitary axis releases endorphins and other neurotransmitters.

A considerable body of evidence supports this line of thinking, particularly as it relates to acupuncture as an anesthetic. What's more, new research indicates that acupuncture releases other substances that trigger different physiological responses, including the following:

- increased white blood cell production, which affects the body's ability to fight infection
- decreased cholesterol and triglycerides (harmful fat particles in the bloodstream), which can reduce the risk of heart disease and related problems
- glucose (blood sugar) and cortisol regulation, which helps the body use energy more efficiently and reduces the risk of diabetes (cortisol is an adrenal hormone that is involved in a number of body processes, including helping us cope with stress)
- regulation and stimulation of serotonin (a neurotransmitter—a chemical produced in the brain and nervous system that facilitates the transfer of information between nerve cells—that is directly related to mood elevation), helping to reduce depression

It appears, then, that acupuncture stimulation produces local effects, acting on nearby nerves to block messages about pain, as well as effects on the structures in the brain that produce endorphins and other brain and body chemicals. The combination of these two effects helps to explain how acupuncture works not only to reduce pain but also to affect the body in a host of other ways.

### The Bioelectromagnetism Theory

The emerging disciplines of bioelectromagnetism and biophysics are providing a new understanding of acupuncture. We now know that within the human body are very low-intensity electromagnetic (EM) fields that signal certain physiological states: EM fields appear to influence biological and circadian rhythms as well as immune and endocrine functions, among others.

External low-intensity EM fields, both natural and man-made, also create specific biological responses. By applying these EM fields in a therapeutic setting, doctors can treat a variety of conditions, including certain bone fractures, chronic pain, and depression and anxiety. Researcher Charles Shang, for instance, has produced studies that show distinct changes in plant and animal tissues within a matter of days following exposure to EM fields.

Other research indicates that there are weak electric fields, naturally occurring forces between atomic particles, that affect the way the body produces and uses calcium. Weak electric fields can inhibit or enhance tumor growth and have been used in a laboratory to regenerate limbs in frogs and starfish. Weak electric fields are difficult to measure due to the larger EM fields of the earth and surrounding elements, as well as man-made fields such as the ones that occur with cell phones, electrical currents, and satellite television. However, more and more research points to their importance in human health and disease.

Some researchers believe that acupuncture works by transmitting electromagnetic signals to adjust physiological functions toward normal. Shang has described "organizing centers," areas that control the oscillatory response in surrounding tissue in areas of low electrical resistance, such as bends in body surfaces, which are precisely the areas in which major acupoints are found. Thus, stimulation at these points with a comparatively weak stimulus can effect large changes in a system.

A different development of this theory involves the Zhang-Popp hypothesis. These researchers sought to explain the fact that acupoints conduct electricity in a unique and identifiable pattern. To do so, they described a model of EM waves created by the many naturally charged particles that are in constant rhythmic motion in the body. These waves have recognizable patterns, which are affected by anatomical structures that form boundaries in the body, such as skin, bones, the linings of tissue (called fascia), and other areas where acupoints are found. The wave patterns are stable but not static, which may explain the phenomenon known as "*qi* movement," the sensation of movement that needling an acupoint can cause, and can be altered by minimal input at the boundary sites.

# Acupuncture in the Twenty-First Century West

Research designed to explain exactly how and why acupuncture works to relieve pain and other ailments continues. It is likely that several of these theories will be shown to have some merit and that a combination of bioelectromagnetic, hormonal, neurological, and even psychological effects derived from acupuncture treatment helps return the body to a state of balance and health. As laid out in the chapters that follow, the richness and complexity of the traditional Chinese medical approach to diagnosis and treatment may never fit neatly into a Western paradigm. For the millions of patients who benefit from acupuncture and related treatments, however, it may well matter less how the treatments work than that they do work—helping people to feel healthier and more vital.

In the meantime, both the National Institutes of Health and the World Health Organization have issued statements confirming the usefulness of acupuncture in the treatment of a wide variety of conditions. According to the NIH's consensus panel of scientists, researchers, and practitioners, who convened in November 1997, acupuncture is an effective treatment for nausea and vomiting caused by surgical anesthesia and cancer chemotherapy, as well as for dental pain experienced after surgery. The panel also found that acupuncture is useful by itself or combined with conventional methods to treat addiction, headaches, menstrual cramps, tennis elbow, fibromyalgia, myofascial pain (pain in muscles and their linings), osteoarthritis, lower back pain, carpal tunnel syndrome, and asthma, as well as in assisting stroke rehabilitation. Part II explores several of these conditions. As preparation, the next chapter provides an overview of the unique diagnostic and treatment methods used in traditional Chinese medicine generally and in acupuncture specifically.

# 4

# TECHNIQUES AND PRACTICES

JUST AS THEORIES OF HEALTH and balance in the East are different from Western views of disease, so too are traditional Chinese methods of diagnosis and treatment. The differences reflect the Chinese medicine view that the external symptoms of diseases are the physiological reflections of internal imbalances in a unified, interconnected energy system. In the West, doctors tend to treat symptoms as if they were localized phenomena that occur independently from the rest of the body, unconnected and discrete.

The two traditions are much different in another way, too. While we in the West attempt to treat all patients having similar symptoms exactly the same—with the same medications or surgical techniques— traditional Chinese practitioners view each patient in a highly individual way, paying close attention to unique physical, psychological, emotional, and intellectual characteristics. Only with this comprehensive information are they able to make a diagnosis, and the treatment that follows is just as unique as the patient is.

If you grew up in the West, you've become used to being treated by Western doctors. Consequently, your first visit to a traditional Chinese practitioner of acupuncture will most likely surprise you; the appointment is likely to be longer, the conversation more personal (if the practitioner speaks English well), and the physical exam more intimate. Your treatments are likely to be less invasive, using fewer (if any) Western medications and subtler approaches such as herbs, breathing exercises, and, of course, acupuncture to reestablish proper balance within the body. For that reason, "results" in the form of symptom relief may arrive more slowly and more subtly than you're used to. In the end, however, you're likely to experience a deeper, longer-lasting, and more fundamental sense of balance and health than you have in the past.

# The Art of Diagnosis

As outlined in Chapter 2, from a traditional Chinese medical perspective, all disease boils down to a disruption of *qi*—its circulation, distribution, function, or production. To diagnose and treat any condition, a practitioner first defines this disruption in terms of the systems that circulate *qi* (the fourteen channels and the organs) and then identifies the illness as a *yin-yang* or Five-Element imbalance.

The method of investigation involves a diagnostic system called the Four Examinations. During your first visit, the practitioner will use these specific examinations to establish a complete picture of your whole system. This process reveals your inherent energy patterns and how your symptoms express them. The Eight Principles further define specific conditions and symptoms in terms of *yin* and *yang*, internal and external, cold and hot, and empty and full. Let's take a closer look.

## *The Four Examinations*

In order to evaluate how energy flows through your body and what may be out of balance, an acupuncturist will apply the Four Examinations: questioning, observing, listening and smelling, and touching. Each method is used in order to discover something that correlates with an imbalance in the *qi*, five elements, and/or *yin-yang* model. Instead of using high technology, or even mid-level technology such as a stethoscope, acupuncturists use their own senses as instruments to measure their patients' various vital signs. The acupuncturist's own experience and powers of observation are the instruments of diagnosis.

*Questioning* As a new acupuncture patient, you may be surprised at how long and how in depth the practitioner questions you. He or she will ask about your medical history, your family's medical history, and your current symptoms and general state of health. The practitioner will also need to know about your hygiene and exercise habits, your sleep patterns and sexual activity, and other lifestyle choices. Additional questions will ascertain your state of mind, your spiritual life, what gives you pleasure, and what causes you stress.

*Observing* You're also likely to be surprised at how the acupuncturist examines you, not only taking your pulse and looking into your eyes, nose, and mouth, as your Western doctor does, but also using the powers of observation in other ways. Often, even as you enter the office and sit down, the practitioner will take note of the way you walk, gesture, and breathe, in order to assess the condition of your overall energy system as well as your sense of self-esteem and the state of your spirit.

He or she also will scan your body, looking for any abnormal signs in your complexion, hair, nails, and skin tone. There are five major skin hues, each of which relates to one of the organ-channel correspondences (refer to "The Five Phases and Correspondences" table in Chapter 2): green—wood/liver; red—fire/heart, yellow—earth/spleen, white—metal/lungs, and blue—water/kidneys. Observing a particular hue to the skin, usually on the temples or around the mouth, directs the practitioner to a potential imbalance affecting the corresponding organ or channel.

In addition, the acupuncturist will take time to examine your tongue. The tongue diagnosis is elaborate and may seem peculiar to the average Westerner visiting a traditional Chinese medicine practitioner. Traditional practitioners observe the tongue's color, size, and shape; whether it is dry or wet; and the coating, or "fur." The fur of the tongue is produced by the process of digestion. The stomach is hot and full of acid, which causes it to emit vapors; these vapors hit the cooler air of the mouth and condense into a coating.

The shape of the tongue generally reflects the body's *yin-yang* balance. Since *yin* refers to the matter, or body, a pointy tongue is considered *yin* deficient, whereas a broader, flabby tongue is *yang* deficient. Because *yin* also refers to fluids, while *yang* refers to heat and dryness, a wet or damp tongue is lacking in *yang*, whereas a dry tongue lacks *yin*. The color of the tongue is important as well. A pale tongue signifies a *yang* deficiency; a tongue that looks red usually means a lack of *yin*. However, a deep red or even purple tongue can denote a stagnant *qi*, which requires correction through acupuncture.

Moreover, the individual areas of the tongue are relevant in the Chinese medicine diagnosis of imbalances. The location of any abnormalities on the tongue or tongue fur directs the practitioner to specific parts of the organ-channel network. Teeth marks, blemishes, concentration of coating, and other signs correlate with particular zones to make the diagnosis. These tongue zones are as follows:

• *Kidney zone* The kidney zone is at the base of the tongue. It corresponds to organs below the navel, including kidneys, large and small intestines, bladder, uterus, ovaries, and testicles. The functions related to the kidney zone include reproduction, elimination, regeneration, and metabolism.

• *Spleen zone* Located in the center of the tongue, the spleen zone corresponds to organs and functions between the diaphragm and navel on the right and left sides, including the stomach, spleen, pancreas, and lower portion of the esophagus and thus digestion and assimilation.

• *Liver zone* The liver zone exists on the sides of the tongue and indicates the state of balance or imbalance in organs on the lateral areas of the body between the diaphragm and navel. These organs and functions include the liver, gallbladder, and spleen and digestion, elimination, and coordination of physiological function.

• *Lung and heart zones*  Located on the tip of the tongue, the lung and heart zones correspond with organs and functions above the diaphragm. The organs include the lungs, heart, esophagus, trachea, nose, ears, mouth, and eyes. The functions involved include respiration, circulation, perception, and communication.

Other tongue signs include the following:

• *Fissured*—indicates dryness of some sort, usually related to digestion; a central fissure can sometimes indicate spinal or back problems.
• *Excessively moist*—indicates dampness.
• *White coat*—indicates excess cold.
• *Yellow coat*—indicates excess heat.
• *Peeled*—indicates some kidney weakness.

Practitioners can spot myriad other signs and symptoms of illness and imbalance by observing the tongue, which is why so much time is spent in such observation during a typical acupuncture examination.

*Listening and Smelling*  Your smell and the way you sound also help a traditional Chinese medicine doctor understand your current state of health. He or she will concentrate on the timbre and tone of your voice, particularly when you're describing subjects with emotional content. Odor is more elusive, but practitioners are trained to notice the subtle odors that we emit, again largely when emotions or interactions are more intense. These odors are distinct from body odor or breath odor and are more akin to the familiar smell of a grandparent. (Western doctors of prior generations were also trained to diagnose illness from certain patient odors, including cases of tuberculosis and diabetes.) The quality of these sounds and odors further guides the practitioner in assessing your state of balance and health, and helps in diagnosing and treating any dysfunction found.

*Touching* You're probably accustomed to your doctor using his or her hands to palpate your body, particularly your abdomen. An acupuncturist, however, will spend much more time feeling your skin and flesh, pressing certain points along your fourteen channels in order to reveal imbalances and disorders within your system. Some practitioners palpate within certain "zones" on the body that signify imbalance in one of the meridians (refer to the "Summary of the Twelve Channels" table in Chapter 2). For instance, tenderness, masses, or thickening of the long muscles of the back would indicate problems in the *tai yang* (small intestine/bladder) meridian.

One of the primary diagnostic techniques is the taking of the pulses. Instead of concentrating on only one radial pulse in the center of your wrist, the acupuncturist takes twelve pulses, found on three points along the radial arteries of the wrists. There are three *yin* pulses and three *yang* pulses that are felt on the right wrist, and the same number of *yin* and *yang* pulses on the left wrist. *Yang* channels are felt more superficially and *yin* channels more deeply on the pulse. However, a practitioner will feel all twelve pulses more superficially than the blood pulsing in the radial artery, since the acupuncture pulses are energy and the blood is solid, or *yin* (and therefore deeper). These twelve pulses reflect the condition of each of the twelve major organ-energy channels. An experienced practitioner can distinguish dozens of different energy patterns in each pulse. He or she looks for differences in the strength of one point in relation to others, which could indicate a problem with the channel or organ that corresponds to that position.

In addition to the Four Examinations, the practitioner will use the Eight Principles to further home in on any imbalances or disruptions in the body's energy system.

## *The Eight Principles*

The Eight Principles help the practitioner determine how *yin* and *yang* are balanced, or out of balance, within the body. The principles are *yin* and *yang*, and three pairs of descriptive factors: cold and hot, empty (deficiency) and full (excess), internal and external. Together, they form a description of an illness by identifying characteristics about it and how the body reacts to it. Hence, a picture or pattern of the disease and its relationships is formed. This is a critical distinction between Western and Chinese medicine. In Western medicine, a disease is seen as discrete. For instance, streptococcus causes sore throat; antibodies to one's joint linings cause rheumatoid arthritis. In Chinese medicine, there are no absolutes. Everything is seen in relationship to the body, to nature, and to other illnesses.

The Eight Principles start with a determination of *yin* and *yang*. Once this diagnosis is made, the other characteristics are defined by the practitioner's asking and answering a series of questions, as follows:

- *Cold* Does warming the area help the problem? Was the problem caused by a cold external influence? Does the person have a cold constitution, one that gets chilled easily and involves a low metabolism?
- *Hot* Is the problem made worse by warming and helped by ice? If it's on the surface, is it warm to the touch? Is this person heat intolerant?
- *Deficiency* Is there a lack of something, such that when energy in the form of movement, heat, or pressure is added, it gets better? Does this problem manifest as a lack of activity?
- *Excess* Is there too much of something, for instance swelling, oozing, redness, or a feeling of fullness and pressure? Does adding energy make it worse? Does rest, lack of movement, and cooling make it better? Is constant activity or movement associated with the problem?

- *Internal* Is the problem inside, deep, diffuse? Which anatomical layer (skin, muscles, viscera) is affected?
- *External* Is the problem on the outside, visible? Is this a problem of the skin, of the connective tissue, or of the superficial muscle?

*Yin* and *yang* are the essentials here, but the other qualities clarify the situation further and lead toward a fuller treatment plan. Once the Eight Principles have been determined, the practitioner can also identify the affected organs or channels and thus describe the pattern more completely.

One of the features of Chinese medicine that fascinates me is the way that we can explain a person's experience of a symptom. For example, suppose you have a pain in your hip. In Western medicine, we would look for a problem of either the tendons or connecting tissue (for instance, bursitis) or simply diagnose arthritis of the joint. In either situation, the treatment is the same: anti-inflammatory medications and perhaps injection or surgery.

However, suppose your pain doesn't come on right away but bothers you more and more as the day wears on. When it hurts, it throbs and feels like a hot poker in your hip, although there is no tenderness. Heat seems to aggravate it a little, but resting it feels great. An acupuncturist would diagnose that as a *yang* pain, since it feels full, throbbing, and hot. It increases when you add energy (movement, pressure from standing and walking, heat). Adding *yin* (rest) helps to balance the yang. This is an excessive *yang* heat pain, probably internal, since it isn't tender. Chances are that the problem lies on the gallbladder (*shao yang*) channel, although pain on the inside of the hip can exist along the liver or spleen channels as well.

Now imagine that your pain feels all right during the day but bothers you throughout the night, causing you a sleepless night. The pain is a deep, dull ache, hard to pinpoint. Using a heating pad helps, as does massage, but you find yourself getting up during the night and "walking it off." This is a *yin*-type pain, and because adding something (movement, massage, heat) helps it, the practitioner would define it as a deficient condition. It feels worse at night (*yin*) and during periods of inactivity (again *yin*).

Or, finally, your condition consists of excruciating pain when you get up in the morning but improves as you move around. Heat and rubbing the joint seem to help as well.

In the first instance—pain that develops gradually—a treatment plan would involve draining or moving the excess *yang*, using points that cool a condition, coupled with rest and perhaps cooling herbs. In the second instance—pain through the night—treatment might include moxa or something else to warm and augment the energy, as well as warming herbs, and movement or exercises. The third instance—excruciating pain in the morning—is more complicated, with both *yang* (worse with movement at first) and *yin* (heat and rubbing help it) characteristics. This is the pain of stagnation in the channels. Sometimes, we call this a "gelling" pain—pain that is liquid as long as there is movement or heat but that gels when it is still. The treatment here is to use points, moxa, and exercises to move the stagnation in the channels.

Internal illnesses tend to be more complex than pain problems. For instance, imagine that you come to the Chinese medicine practitioner with bloating, diarrhea, and indigestion (let's assume that your doctor has ruled out serious illness). The acupuncturist would use the Four Examinations to determine the problem. He or she would *question* you extensively about the nature of your diet, the situations and timing that bring on the symptoms, past illnesses and history, emotional factors involved, and many other pieces of information. You report that soup feels good but that drinking carbonated beverages and eating ice cream bother your stomach a lot. You are often tired, and you have little appetite. Your belly is so bloated that you have to loosen your clothing. Applying a hot water bottle at night helps. Your bowel movements are loose and gassy.

The practitioner will *listen* for evidence of a significant vocal quality, such as weeping (the sound of the large intestine/metal imbalance) or singing (a spleen/earth sound). Let us say there is a slightly whiny, modulated quality to your voice. He or she will *observe* your tongue, finding it to be puffy and pale, with a wet, white, slightly sticky coating. The acupuncturist will *palpate* your belly, perhaps finding the middle area colder than the others and some tenderness around the umbilicus. Your pulse will merit a lot of attention, perhaps with the middle right (earth) position feeling somewhat puffy and weak.

The diagnosis here is a deficiency of the spleen (earth) *yang* energy. Deficiency is evident in the tongue, the pulse, and the tiredness. Spleen involvement is indicated in the cold palpated in the spleen area of the abdomen, by the tongue, and by the presentation of symptoms. There is lack of heat and lack of *yang*. The treatment will involve warming the channels, warming the belly, a diet of warm and simple foods, and perhaps some *qi gong* exercises and herbs to raise spleen *qi*.

Thus, the practitioner utilizes the Four Examinations and Eight Principles to create a highly individual, highly focused treatment plan.

# Treatment: The Eightfold Path Toward Health

As you might imagine after gaining an understanding of the Eastern view of health and its unique diagnostic technique, treatment within this context also differs distinctly from the Western model. The primary difference between the two approaches is that the traditional Chinese way is a holistic one that treats the whole body system, while we in the West tend to focus only on the part of the body where overt symptoms appear. The results of such treatments often reflect those same biases, with Eastern remedies leading to a rebalancing of the entire body and thus longer-lasting and deeper health. Western remedies tend to be quick—and often short-term—fixes that bring rapid relief of complaints but never address the underlying dysfunction that allowed the condition to emerge.

Traditional Chinese medicine focuses on eight treatment methods, also known as the Eightfold Path or the Tree of Health. The methods are acupuncture, Chinese herbal medicine, diet and nutrition, *qi gong* exercise, *qi gong* breathing, meditation, massage and acupressure, and right living (also known as wisdom). These practices range from the strictly physical (massage, diet) to the spiritual. It is important to remember that Chinese medicine originated from Taoist, spiritual concepts, and purity of thought and behavior is seen as leading to the highest form of a healthy mind, body, and spirit. These eight methods are detailed in Part II; the remainder of this chapter gives you an overview.

### Acupuncture: The Finer Points

Unlike a pill or surgical procedure, a series of acupuncture treatments neither provides instant results nor produces discrete effects on a single symptom, organ, or system. Instead, the goal of treatment, over time, is to reestablish balance throughout the entire body, and it does so without causing "side effects" that are expected with most Western treatments and are so detrimental to general health. In fact, the idea that a treatment for one imbalance could be called successful if it can resolve one symptom only by triggering an imbalance in another part of the body is contrary to Eastern concepts of health and healing.

Throughout the body, located along the fourteen channels, are hundreds of acupoints, areas that can be stimulated to enhance and manipulate the flow of *qi* and the functions of the organ networks. In selecting the appropriate points for treatment, an acupuncturist considers the following options (among others):

• *Location*  A point may be chosen on the channel nearest the site of the problem. In some cases, an acupuncturist will use a local point close to the site of the symptom—one outside the nostril in the case of nasal congestion, for instance, or points in the vicinity of a painful ankle sprain.

• *Points with channel-based functions* Some points are used to open flow into a meridian, or to allow energy from one channel into another. For instance, a deficiency of the spleen channel may be treated by using a point on the inside of the foot, which is called a junction, or *luo* point, because it joins the spleen and stomach channels and allows them to come into balance. One patient of mine broke her ankle and was obliged to use crutches, after which she developed fatigue and insomnia. My examination revealed that she had blocked the entry point to the heart channel, located in the armpit. Needling this point restored her energy and good sleep.

• *Points with* yin-yang *or Eight Principles functions* Various points are known to drain dampness, to cool off heat, or to build *qi*. Some points are used in combination to obtain certain results. For instance, two stomach points on the leg are known to build blood, while another stomach point nearby gets rid of dampness.

• *Points known to rebalance the five elements* There are five points on each of the twelve arm and leg channels that correspond to each of the five phases. These points act as links and passages in the body's energy system, which is why needling one of them may affect the balance of them all. For example, when the wood energy becomes stuck (as it often is), it cannot feed the fire according to the creative cycle. Using "tonification" (strengthening) points on the fire channels (found on the forearm) moves energy from wood to fire, thereby balancing both channels.

• *Points that act directly on the organ* Some points, particularly on the back along the bladder channel, affect the corresponding organ. There are also some channels, the Distinct Meridians, that are accessed by points on the fourteen channels and that act on the organs. For instance, a practitioner might help to treat a bladder infection by using Distinct Meridian points on the bladder and kidney channels, or by using a special point, called a *"shu"* or Associated Effect point. This point is on the lower back, and affects the bladder.

After choosing the appropriate points, the practitioner inserts very thin needles rapidly through the skin to a depth of about one-fourth inch to two inches or more. The depth depends on a variety of factors, including the patient's size and the part of the body involved. The needles are left in place for a time lasting from a few seconds up to an hour; the average is about twenty minutes, although some treatment styles do not leave needles in at all.

A practitioner may use other methods apart from needle insertion. The most common of these is moxibustion, which uses focused heat generated by burning moxa, dried leaves of the Chinese herb mugwort. Cupping, which employs vacuum suction with glass globes or bamboo jars, is another technique used to manipulate the flow of *qi* through the body.

*Microsystems: The Art of Acupuncture Expands*  There are even more uses for the remarkable little acupuncture needles than the "standard" acupuncture treatments you've just been reading about, most significantly a group of techniques known as microsystems. Microsystems are organized around the theory that the entire body may be mapped in a single area, such as the ear or the scalp, with each location on the map representing a different part of the body and different functions. This map, sometimes called a humunculus, is distorted in its picture of the human form. It is upside down, and certain portions of the body (head, hands, and feet, particularly) are much larger proportionally.

The most widely known microsystem is ear acupuncture, sometimes called auriculotherapy. Auriculotherapy as it is practiced today is not ancient Chinese in origin, although ancient texts do mention that acupuncture channels may cross the ear. Modern auriculotherapy actually originated with Dr. Paul Nogier of France in the early 1950s. Nogier charted points on the ear that correspond to areas of the body and began to publish charts and treatment protocols. These publications spread to Germany, Japan, and finally China, where they became widely incorporated into the Chinese medicine teaching programs.

In particular, many practitioners used these points in studies of surgical anesthesia. More recently, the work of Dr. Bruce Pomeranz and others has helped clarify the connection between ear points and pain control by identifying natural pain-relief substances called endorphins. Endorphins work somewhat like opioids (pharmaceutical painkillers) in the body and can be released by the stimulation of certain ear points, among other acupoints. In addition to managing pain, practitioners often use auriculotherapy to treat addiction (discussed in Chapter 6). Asthma, digestive problems, myriad gynecological complaints, and even attention deficit–hyperactivity disorder in children may also be treated using this therapy.

Other acupuncture systems have sprung up similarly, as physicians have discovered these correspondences in other areas of the body. One type of acupuncture, used for decades in Chinese practice, concentrates on the scalp, and areas corresponding to the areas of the brain have been used successfully in the treatment of brain injuries and other conditions. A more recent system, developed by Dr. Toshikatsu Yamamoto and called Yamamoto New Scalp Acupuncture, is being used in Japan and the United States to address musculoskeletal problems. Facial acupuncture, utilizing specific points on the face to treat parts of the body, has been used in medical conditions such as abdominal pain and sinus inflammation, as well as in addiction treatments. Recently, a microsystem using ocular (eye) diagnosis and points around the orbit has been described. A system of foot points can be used to treat parts of the body as well. This system, called reflexology, involves massage of the various foot points rather than the use of needles.

A Korean system of hand acupuncture popularized in the United States by Tae Woo Yoo utilizes points on the hands to treat the various meridians. In this system, Chinese medicine strategies are employed, but instead of treating the body points, corresponding points on the hands are needled, usually with tiny, two- to four-millimeter needles or with small metal press balls, tiny pellets held onto the point with small bandages. In this way, treatments that are difficult to negotiate, such as point combinations on the front and back together or points in sensitive places of the body, can be easily addressed by treating the hand. Children can also be treated more easily in this manner.

Some modern acupuncturists use low-level electrical currents to stimulate acupoints. A small electrical device is attached with alligator clips to the needles, and a current is pulsed through them. Many scientific studies involving acupuncture use this method, which is called *electroacupuncture*.

When you visit a practitioner for the first time, discuss the acupuncture techniques he or she uses most often. If you're interested in exploring auriculotherapy or another microsystem, see the Appendix for a listing of resources.

## *Chinese Herbal Medicine*

The use of herbs is an essential part of traditional Chinese medicine. In fact, herbal medicine—particularly that practiced within traditional Chinese medicine—is the most ancient form of health care in the world. Herbs help reorganize the body constituents (*qi*, blood, and body fluids) within the meridians and the internal organs, for instance to help unstick *qi* that's blocked or to compensate for a lack of moisture in the lungs. In addition, they can help the body adjust to the impact of any external forces, as in strengthening an immune system in preparation for the cold of winter.

In general, Chinese herbal medicine uses multiple herbs in combinations. Most often, the individual herbs are combined to maximize their effects on the body's energy balance. A common formula usually includes two or three main herbs, as well as assisting herbs (mostly to modify the harsher effects of the main herbs or to direct the treatment toward a specific meridian or organ), and some herbs to harmonize the combination and make it palatable. When the practitioner individualizes a combination of herbs, other herbs are generally added for specific effects on symptoms such as sleep, pain, or inflammation.

The resulting combination of herbs generally has few side effects and frequently can treat problems in ways that the individual herbs cannot. One common Chinese combination of herbs, *suan zao ren*, has been demonstrated in clinical studies to have sedating effects equal to prescription sleep medications, but none of the individual herbs in the formula demonstrates any of these sleep-producing properties on its own.

For an example of how a practitioner might prescribe a Chinese herbal formula, consider a patient of mine who was nearing menopause. Her menstrual periods had become lighter, she was feeling more tired than usual, and her skin was noticeably drier. In addition, she was beginning to experience hot flashes, most frequently at night and interfering with her already light sleep. In Chinese medicine terms, she had deficient blood (literally, and also a depletion of the *yin* of her body, which is associated with the physical or blood portion of the energy).

Because of the lack of the *yin*/blood with its cooling, moistening, and anchoring properties, she was having symptoms of heat moving upward, of dryness, of restlessness and exhaustion, and of a worsening of symptoms in the *yin* (night) time. The basic formula was a "blood-building" formula (remember, this blood deficiency does not have to do with anemia, but more with the quality that is called blood in Chinese medicine). These herbs tend to go to the spleen (which builds the blood) and the liver (which moves it). In addition, some kidney-building herbs address the deficiency of *yin*. This formula, a time-honored one, is called eight precious or women's precious formula. To further deal with the sleep problems, the formula might also contain herbs that "calm the spirit," such as biota and polygala, along with certain herbs that cool down the heat associated with a *yin* lack, such as philodendron or anemarhena.

A Chinese herbalist may prepare formulas for both internal and external application. Internal preparations may include any of the following:

• **Raw herbs** Commonly served as broths or decoctions (extracts made from roots and barks), the herbs are cooked in water for minutes or hours, after which the liquid is strained; it is used for a one- to three-day period.

• *Powders* These mixtures of pulverized raw herbs are usually taken with water.

• *Capsules* Powdered herbs are pressed into capsules to be swallowed.

• *Tablets or pills* More frequently, practitioners are prescribing herbal remedies that are already patented and in pill form. Although the options for individualizing a treatment are lost, the advantages include convenience, confidence that the patient is receiving what has been prescribed (quality control), and the ability to modify doses. In the foregoing example, I might have given the patient a patented "women's precious" pill plus another one for kidney *yin* and lessening heat, or perhaps a more general *yin*-building pill and another to help control sleep.

• *Extracts or tinctures* This is another more modern way of controlling doses and better measuring what a patient is receiving. It is more convenient than raw herbs, but not everyone likes the taste of herbal tinctures.

The various ways that herbal treatments are given externally include the following:

• Pastes
• Ointments
• Suppositories
• Vaginal douches and washes

## Diet and Nutrition

Fourteen centuries ago, the Chinese physician Sun Ssu-mao wrote, "The truly good physician . . . first treats the patient with food; only when food fails does he resort to drugs." Sun Ssu-mao had a kindred spirit in his much earlier Western colleague Hippocrates, who wrote, "Thy food be thy medicine."

Today, we all seem to be striving to maintain a "balanced diet." Here in the West, we take that to mean a combination of foods that have a proportional amount of protein, carbohydrates, fat, vitamins, and minerals. In the East, the concept of "balanced" is much richer, more elaborate, and more integral to the way the body functions. What represents a balanced diet in the East is a highly individual matter, depending entirely on the person's unique physical, spiritual, and intellectual makeup. A traditional Chinese medical practitioner will select food for a patient by its correspondence with the individual's innate patterns as well as the person's conditions or symptoms at a given time. Generally speaking, someone with a cold, dry condition, for instance, should eat warm, moisturizing food; someone with a hot, damp condition would be prescribed cool, drying food.

A Chinese nutritionist may also prescribe foods in order to protect someone from external environmental influences that would disrupt the internal *yin-yang* balance. In a very cold, damp, and overcast climate (a *yin* climate), you may want to eat warm, stimulating *yang* foods in order to better protect yourself. Finally, all food is associated with one of the five elements. This correspondence determines the food's affinities for various organ networks in the body. One of the most obvious relationships, when it comes to food, is the five flavors (see page 27).

Clearly, diet is an important treatment method, especially in combination with others such as acupuncture and meditation. In fact, because food has its own energy and medicinal properties, a smart practitioner will always make dietary recommendations, if only to avoid having a patient's diet interfere with the actions of herbs or the therapeutic value of acupuncture.

Some aspects of Chinese dietary therapy are quite different from what a Western nutritionist might recommend. For instance, food is almost always cooked, since raw foods are thought to put a strain on the spleen. A prescription for digestive problems might include warm soups and stews. Meanwhile, our Western diets are filled with "cold" foods, from sweets to snack foods to sandwiches and salads, and washed down by soda; from a Chinese medicine perspective, it's no wonder our culture is beset with irritable bowel and other digestive problems.

Other dietary suggestions may be more familiar to you. Hot, pungent foods (which have an affinity for the lungs and metal) help treat a mucus-producing respiratory problem (think here of chicken soup), while salty foods are used for fatigue and dehydration, since they aid the kidneys.

## Qi Gong *Exercise and* Qi Gong *Breathing*

As mentioned in Chapter 2, the word *qi* has many meanings, including not only "energy" but also "breath" and "air." The word *gong* means "exercise" or "skill." *Qi gong*, then, means "the skill of breath and energy control," and the exercises involved develop and require these skills. Although technically occupying two different stretches of the Eightfold Path Toward Health, *qi gong* breathing and *qi gong* exercise are almost impossible to separate in a discussion, since they are part and parcel of one another.

One of the prime benefits of practicing *qi gong* exercises is an increase in one's energy reserves and daily energy levels. According to Chinese theory, the body stores *qi* in an area known as the Sea of Energy (called *dan tien* in Chinese, *hara* in Japanese), located just below and behind the navel. *Qi gong* exercises act to increase the reserves as well as to guide energy circulation through all fourteen channels and thus to all of the organs in the body. But that's not all. *Qi gong* works on three levels: the body, the breath, and the mind. To perform the simple, elegant, yet demanding exercises, one must concentrate on all three. First, the body will move rhythmically, bathing the organs and channels with energy. The mind will be engaged as well, not in activity, but in quiet concentration; *qi gong* engenders mental tranquility and serenity, which further helps the flow of *qi*.

But it is the breath, or more accurately, focused breathing, that lies at the heart of *qi gong*'s power. Specifically, learning *qi gong* means learning deep abdominal breathing, which uses the diaphragm, the muscle that lies at the base of the chest cavity and atop the abdominal cavity. In deep abdominal breathing, the diaphragm descends toward the abdominal organs when one inhales and rises back into the chest cavity when one exhales. Breathing deeply in this way not only massages the internal organs but also increases blood flow by boosting upward the flow of blood to the heart, which then pumps it out into the rest of the body.

In Chinese medicine terms, the breath comes from the heavens and therefore bathes us in spiritual energy. Exhaling lets go of any "bad energy"—toxic thoughts or feelings and tensions that have built up. Think of sighing deeply and the releasing sensation that it gives. In fact, one of the common *qi gong* exercises for the lungs is to sigh loudly and rapidly, throwing the hands down at the same time and letting go of tensions and stress, while making room for freshness and spiritual cleansing.

The many forms of *qi gong* include martial arts practices such as *karate* and *tai kwan do*, as well as meditation techniques in the Taoist tradition. (Perhaps you've seen people practicing these slow, controlled movements early in the morning in your local park.) In China, hundreds of older people practice a slow, dancelike *qi gong* called *tai chi* each morning, to maintain their vitality and flexibility. *Qi gong* movement and breathing systems are simple, universal in their applications, and conducive to good physical health and mental well-being. (Chapters 8 and 9 delve further into these concepts.)

## Meditation

Meditation is another form of *qi gong*. In fact, it is the highest form of this ancient practice. Meditation influences the flow of *qi* from the highest level of being, the spirit, and allows someone who practices medita-

tion to take in *qi* from nature and from the heavens. The act of meditation also clears the mind, which allows *qi* to flow unobstructed
throughout the fourteen channels and the organ networks.

Meditation involves little more than—as the Chinese put it—"sitting still and doing nothing." This is harder than it appears, however,
because the goal of this effort is to attain such a clarity and stillness of
mind that one can quiet two particularly noisy aspects of oneself: the
intellect and the emotions. Indeed, traditional Chinese theory considers an overactive intellect and high-strung emotions to be forms of disease and disorder.

Dr. Herbert Benson of Harvard Medical School has described
something called the relaxation response, which is the body's physiological response to meditation. The basis of this physiological response
is akin to the Chinese medicine concept of *yin* and *yang*. The *"yang"*
neurological function of the body is governed by the sympathetic nervous system, commonly called the fight-or-flight response. Prolonged
exposure to the reaction of this system, which is activated by stress, leads
to a wearing down of the body's tissues, as well as to a depletion of neurotransmitters, resulting in depression, and to an increase in chronic
conditions such as back pain, heart disease, and immune weakness.

To counteract this, we have a *"yin"* response called the parasympathetic nervous system. As Benson and others have shown, meditation is
one of the best ways of releasing this response. The long-term results
of meditation and the relaxation response are lower blood pressure, less
stress-related illness, a calmer and more satisfied mental state, and a
healthy immunity. Long before the physiology was explained, Chinese
medicine practitioners understood the importance of this calming state
in the path toward greater health (discussed in Chapter 6).

## Massage and Acupressure

Areas called zones, located on the surface, match the fourteen channels
that run inside our bodies. Tiny meridians run into the skin and mus-

cle tissue from the major channels, so that energy moves through these tissues as well. Therefore, any blockage of the major channels is transported to the muscles and subcutaneous tissues, as well as to the skin. Likewise, injuries that scar and penetrate these tissues can affect the flow of *qi* in the meridians. Tightness of muscles and other injuries alter the *qi* as well.

Massaging the superficial tissues, therefore, has a profound effect on the overall energy. Of the several systems of massage in Chinese medicine, the most distinctive is acupressure (or *shiatsu*, from the Japanese word). In this system, the practitioner massages acupoints on the surface of the body, sometimes applying enough pressure to affect the meridians themselves. The goal is similar to that of acupuncture. A good acupressurist can move or redirect *qi* and treat a variety of physical ailments. Self-acupressure is becoming an increasingly popular form of self-care. Frequently, I will send my patients home with a drawing of several points to massage for certain problems. For instance, pressure on spleen 6 (on the inner leg) can help to alleviate menstrual cramps, and pericardium 6 (on the inside surface of the arm) is sometimes useful in treating nausea. As noted, the system of acupressure that focuses on treating points on the hands and feet is known as reflexology.

Other forms of massage are also useful in the holistic approach of Chinese medicine. In a form sometimes called *qi gong* massage, a practitioner might work the long muscles of the body, seeking to relax the muscles and move the *qi* that has become blocked. Some forms of massage work specifically on scar tissue, looking to soften the scar and allow greater flow of blood and energy through the damaged area. (Chapter 5 has more on this subject.)

A particularly specialized form called *tuina* is a gentle type of massage that uses repetitive strokes in the areas of the body where energy might be blocked. Much gentler than acupuncture, *tuina* is a common form of treatment for infants and children, since children's blockages are newer and don't tend to be as stubborn to remedy. Frequently, parents can be taught to perform the simple movements on their children. I have shown a number of parents the *tuina* massage technique to help their children with sleep problems, as well as other massage movements to strengthen an infant's weakened respiratory system.

## Right Living

Chinese medicine began as part of Taoism, the spiritual system of the East based on balance of body, mind, and spirit. The Tao literally is "the way of life." That way comprises all of the other pathways, including healthy breathing, movement and energy exercises, balanced diet, massage and other techniques to keep the body and mind vital, and a lifestyle of moderation and balance. Thousands of years ago, in *The Yellow Emperor's Classic of Internal Medicine*, Qi Po, the book's narrator and teacher, laid out this pathway toward greater health and longer life for his royal pupil, the Yellow Emperor.

More than this, following the Tao means a healthy, honorable way of being in the world. It means being charitable and kind, acting rationally and avoiding impetuousness, and pursuing the higher road in all situations. The *I Ching*, or "Book of Changes," which we think of as a fortune-telling tool, is actually a guide toward finding the "right" actions at all times. According to ancient Chinese belief, all of the consequences of how people live their lives are the results of their physical, mental, and spiritual pursuits. Therefore, a life devoted to the healthy and balanced expression of these pursuits would result in vitality, longevity, and equanimity.

Part II takes you deeper into the world of the five elements to reveal how this natural view of the body and of the natural rhythms of health and healing may explain some common medical conditions. You'll also learn about effective and safe treatments from the Eightfold Path Toward Health.

# THE FIVE-ELEMENT THEORY

As you'll see in this next series of chapters, the Five-Element theory embedded in traditional Chinese therapy is a highly personal and individualized one. A practitioner trained in the fine art of diagnosis within this framework will observe certain personality traits, ways of movement, emotional expressions, and patterns of symptoms in a patient. These observations allow the practitioner to determine what type of person the patient most resembles within the Five-Element theory. By doing so, the practitioner is able to both anticipate patterns of disease and focus treatment options in more specific ways. As you read these chapters, you're sure to see aspects of yourself and the people you love reflected in the five elements.

5

# WOOD
## Free and Easy Wanderer

WOOD ENERGY IS THE ENERGY of spring, of birth and new growth. When a sprout pops through the ground in early spring, it is an act of drive and single-mindedness. The energy of that sprout is focused; it has a direction, a goal, and it will push through anything in its path or find a way around it. Each spring, my herb garden stages a demonstration of wood energy at work in the environment. There is a race to push through the ground and to claim space. One year, the spearmint gains the advantage by sending tentacles into nearby patches of space and rooting. The thyme gathers its small leaves about itself and, using its bulk, pushes into gaps between the mint projections. Meanwhile, the comfrey pushes upward, claiming the air above the other herbs with its prickly, fanlike leaves. It is a battle for territory, each plant looking to move upward and outward. Just as a preadolescent child is a blur of activity, movement, and testing of limits and boundaries, so too is wood energy always looking for boundaries and, once it finds them, will push against them.

Wood is about creation and creativity. That creativity can be a spark of understanding, or a rush of ideas and insights that mirrors the explosive energy of wood in other ways. The wood mind is full of ideas, sometimes single-minded to the point of excluding other things. It is wood energy that gives the burst of artistic activity. This energy is Archimedes shouting "Eureka!" as he sat in his bathtub thinking of a way to prove that his emperor's crown was made of pure gold. It is the fury with which Michelangelo attacked his marble, barely stopping to eat or sleep.

If you're someone characterized by wood energy, you may be domineering, ambitious, and competitive. Nurturing interpersonal relationships through conversation is not your highest priority: when you talk, you talk about specific subjects concerning your life, or about ideas, but you're not a sympathetic listener like your earth energy counterpart or even a playful conversationalist like your fire brethren. You like getting your point across: "This is what *I* think," you tend to say. Anger may be your strongest emotion, but as long as you keep it in balance, expressing your anger is healthy for you. Just as thunder clears the air, so too do outbursts of your inner thoughts of frustration or stress help you maintain your health and inner balance.

This is not to say that all people with wood energy are angry all the time. It is just as common to find those with wood energy unable to express their anger directly. Here in the West, we call these people passive-aggressive, but in Chinese medicine, such behavior represents blocked or stuck wood energy. In my practice, I sometimes elicit this trait by asking what the patient's experiences were with other doctors. If the response is something like, "None of them had any #$&@^*&# idea what was wrong with me!" then I'll suspect that there is stuck wood energy. This is particularly likely if the patient expresses other indirect anger or disgust, such as in reference to the parking outside my office, the need to take so many pills, or difficulties with coworkers.

A healthy wood energy, in contrast, is characterized by a clear and hopeful vision of the future. In fact, the exit point of the liver channel

is called the "gate of hope," and several points on the gallbladder channel refer to vision: "eye window" is a point on the head; "bright and
clear" is the junction (*luo*) point on the leg. The source point of the gallbladder, which sums up the essence of the channel, is called "wilderness
mound." Although some interpret the name of the point literally to refer
to the lateral ankle bone that lies beside it, others see in the name an
image of a high place that gives vision and perspective to one's life.
Vision itself is a wood energy function, and the eye is related to wood:
in the poetic world of Chinese medicine, the gallbladder and liver channels can be used to address problems of physical vision as well as the
inability to visualize a clear and promising future for oneself.

## Wood Energy in Health and Disease

Believe it or not, two furniture upholsterers made medical history in the
early 1960s. The workers were repairing the couches of a pair of cardiologists as well as those of other specialists in the doctors' suite of
offices. The upholsterers astutely noticed that the fronts of the chairs in
the cardiologists' waiting room were heavily worn, indicating that the
cardiology patients had persistently sat forward on their seats, as if they
were anxious. In contrast, the couches of other physicians, including
dermatologists and gastroenterologists, were worn at their rears, as if
their patients had relaxed back into their seats while calmly waiting for
their doctors. Thus was identified what would become a very modern
idea about people with heart conditions: also known as type A personalities, those with cardiac problems tended to be tenser, more impatient,
and more stressed than their noncardiac counterparts.

In my practice, my receptionist has learned to recognize the people
with stuck wood energy. They might be upset with the procedure at the
front desk or indignant when told that their insurance doesn't cover acupuncture. They bristle when they are kept waiting. Although I do my
best to be punctual, if I walk into the room even five or ten minutes late,

they look first at their watches and then slowly up at me, putting me at somewhat of a psychological disadvantage. As I review their symptoms and history, they present the information in a manner that suggests that someone (me, a former doctor, a boss) has messed up in some way, bringing them to this situation. It is a sense of frustration that tends to "push against" others, leaving people wondering if they did something wrong. But there's nothing wrong, just the natural quality of the wood energy, looking for something to push against.

This is how wood energy looks when there is a problem: frustrated. Again, while the primary emotion of wood energy is anger, it is not necessarily explosive anger. More commonly, the emotion associated with the wood element is a constant dissatisfaction, a sense of being trapped and limited, and of pushing against those limitations. Sudden winds or climate changes may also affect wood energy. A healthy wind brings freshness: think of opening the window to the gentle spring breezes, cleansing and fragrant. Likewise, a certain kind of unpredictability can signify free-moving wood, be it the creative freshness of an actor's improvisation or the graceful flexibility of an athlete.

Centuries ago, Chinese medical practitioners too had identified the type A personality. They described it as a wood energy imbalance. According to the *sheng* or creative cycle as described in Chapter 2, the liver, which is the *yin* organ of wood energy, feeds the heart. When liver energy becomes stuck or stagnant, the heart will often fail to receive the energy it needs, and disease can easily result. In women, this imbalance often causes menstrual dysfunction, which is discussed later in this chapter.

When the *yang* organ of the wood energy, the gallbladder, becomes imbalanced, the muscles, bones, and joints can fail to function in health and balance. Headaches, a result of both muscular tension and emotional frustration, may result as well. Of course, both organs work together with the rest of the five elements, so that the ultimate cause of symptoms can lie anywhere.

## *Wood* Yin: *The Free and Easy Wanderer*

The liver is the *yin* organ of wood energy, and it represents the principles of movement and organization. Much as the sprout must have a clear plan of where it is going (up and out of the earth), so too does the body. The liver, known as the "planner," governs the movement of the body, mind, and spirit. When the liver energy is healthy and in balance, it keeps blood, energy, and emotions flowing. The liver is also an integral part of the creative spirit; when it is functioning well, you're able to communicate well and express yourself creatively. The liver channel, along with the pericardium, is part of a greater channel called *jue yin*. It begins on the inner side of the great toe and ascends the inside surface of the leg and into the groin. It ends at the bottom of the ribs, on the front of the body. Internal branches circle the genitals and move through the abdomen to the liver. (See Figure 1 on the following page and Figure 6 on page 140.)

From a Western perspective, the liver is responsible for filtering, detoxifying, and replenishing the body. It also helps to synthesize protein from the food that is consumed, which enables the body to build and repair muscle. In Chinese medicine, the liver energy has a particular significance in gynecology. The liver governs the cyclical movement of blood, so the menstrual cycle is intimately connected with wood. When the liver works well, the cycles are regular, and the transition from one stage of the cycle to another is smooth. In fact, the liver is responsible for the smooth movement of physiological and natural cycles generally, including sleep and day-to-night cycles. When wood energy is imbalanced, insomnia and other sleep disturbances may occur.

Unfortunately, the energy of the liver easily becomes blocked. As discussed, frustration and anger may disrupt the function of the organ, as may something physical that is blocking the energy in the lower abdomen and pelvis, such as scarring from surgery or muscle spasms. In addition, if you eat a poor diet or become depleted of nutrients for any

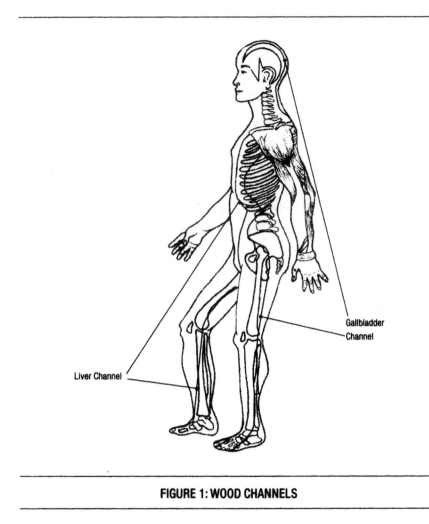

Gallbladder
Channel

Liver Channel

**FIGURE 1: WOOD CHANNELS**

reason, the blood may become sluggish. Infection or inflammation in
the pelvis may also cause liver imbalance.

Wherever there is stagnant energy, pain and inflammation result.
In women, this stagnation often leads to endometriosis or painful menstrual cramps. Premenstrual syndrome (PMS), with its pelvic discomfort and emotional symptoms, is another symptom of stagnant liver
energy. Infections that turn into pelvic inflammatory disease (PID)

cause heat and inflammation in the pelvis. Similarly, irregular cycles and infertility, especially when accompanied by cramping, can be a wood energy problem. The "free and easy wanderer," a common herbal formula used to treat stuck wood energy, describes the goal of a wood treatment: to relax and soften the liver energy.

## *Wood* Yang: *The Wilderness Mound*

Because the gallbladder is a *yang* organ, it controls the more superficial and active tissues, specifically the ligaments and tendons. These connective tissues hold bones together and hold the muscles to the bones. Proper musculoskeletal function requires soft, fluid motion of these tissues, and this, like flexibility in general, largely depends on wood energy.

The gallbladder channel starts next to the eye and runs across the side of the head, into the trapezius muscle on the top of the shoulder, and down the flank. It then goes down the long muscle at the side of the leg, the fascia lata, and down the tibia on the outside of the foreleg and through the outer ankle to the fourth toe. (See Figure 1 earlier in this chapter.)

Problems with the gallbladder energy manifest themselves in tightness and spasms of the muscles, and sprains and strains of tendons and ligaments. Flexibility decreases, and the musculoskeletal system becomes more prone to injury. Frequently, the injuries and tightness lie over the gallbladder or its greater channel, the *shao yang* (gallbladder/triple heater), but most lack of flexibility or tightness involves the wood energy. Tension headaches may also result from a disruption of gallbladder energy, particularly as the channel crosses the temples and the top of the skull.

I have many wood imbalance patients in my practice. While it's impossible to generalize, they do share certain traits. One category of wood energy patient includes people who are aggressive in both their business and personal lives and who appear to have difficulty forming close emotional relationships. They frequently hold jobs that use their organizational skills, such as office manager, personal assistant, or executive. Running or another active exercise is important to this type; if they can't run or ski or row, they're miserable. Women in this category often report having pelvic pain, such as endometriosis; headaches; and premenstrual syndrome.

Another patient pattern, male or female, is someone who seems to be directionless and drifting in jobs and relationships. Even the voice seems to lack power (called "lack of shout" in Chinese medicine). People in this category frequently report having headaches, insomnia, or fatigue. And yet, they have an edge underneath their exhaustion. Sometimes, it feels as if they are daring me to make them better.

# Treating Wood Energy Imbalance

Do you find yourself feeling constantly tense and irritated? Is your life plagued by muscle aches and strains? Are headaches common? If you're a woman, do you suffer from PMS or other menstrual disorders? Have you had trouble sleeping? If you have any of these symptoms, your alternative practitioner will concentrate on bringing your body back into balance by using acupuncture and other aspects of the Eightfold Path Toward Health as explained in Chapter 4. Several studies attest to the effectiveness of acupuncture in alleviating the conditions commonly caused by a disruption of liver energy, particularly PMS and tension headaches. Dietary measures may also help to restore balance and health in this pathway.

However, of the five elements, wood is one of the most vulnerable to stress and stress-related disorders. If your wood is imbalanced, it's likely that you become so busy, so intensely involved in your daily life, that you forget to relax, to slow down and take time to carve out moments of peace for your body and mind. You're also likely to have tense muscles and an overactive fight-or-flight response. Given these circumstances, your practitioner will probably suggest meditation and relaxation techniques to help bring your body back into balance and flexibility exercises to combat all the muscle and joint tightness that has developed along with the stress. Many underlying physical and emotional problems may naturally resolve as this process of relaxation proceeds.

## Qi Gong *Massage: Working Through the Stress*

For centuries, healers from virtually every culture around the world have used the power of touch as a method of curing illness and relieving pain. From both Eastern and Western perspectives, massage helps to stimulate healing and promote the free flow of energy through the body and mind. Massage can reduce muscle tension, improve circulation, and relax an overstressed, overburdened nervous system.

There are dozens of massage techniques that can help someone with the kind of pain and inflexibility that results from an imbalance of wood energy. These include a score of Western forms of therapeutic massage along with several Eastern techniques. *Shiatsu*, which utilizes strong finger pressure on specific acupoints, is especially helpful in easing headaches and muscle soreness, as well as improving posture by realigning the spine.

*Qi gong* massage is the name given to body work performed by experienced *qi gong* practitioners. In this treatment, the muscles of the body are massaged with long strokes. Oils are sometimes used, and the massage resembles athletic or Swedish massage. The chief difference is that the massage strokes are performed along the pathways of the meridians that run through the muscle. In addition, the practitioner uses his or her own *qi*, as well as hands, to move energy through the channels. In this way, a trained practitioner can accomplish the same effect as acupuncture, unblocking stagnation of energy and softening the muscles. This is critical in treating wood energy, since stagnation is the most frequent

form of imbalance, and the muscles are common sites for this stagnation. Some *qi gong* masters can actually move energy through a patient's
channels by holding their hands lightly over the person's body!


## Treating Menstrual Disorders

Premenstrual syndrome, excessively heavy or cramping periods, and
pelvic pain from endometriosis or pelvic inflammatory disease (usually
triggered by infection with bacteria or viruses) are common problems
in women everywhere. In the West, such conditions have a variety of
causes, but almost all relate to disruptions in the balance of female hormones involved in the menstrual cycle. Endometriosis, for instance, is
a process in which estrogen-sensitive tissue implants outside the uterus.
At each menstrual period, the tissue cramps and bleeds, often causing
intolerable pain. Doctors treat this condition and most other hormone-
related menstrual disorders with analgesics, hormone medication, and/or
surgery.

Within the Chinese medical paradigm, these conditions are considered wood energy problems. The wood *yin* organ, the liver, is responsible for moving the blood, and when blood doesn't move well, it either
clumps up and forms masses (fibroids or ovarian tumors), stagnates and
becomes tender and painful (PID, endometriosis), or causes symptoms
of "stuckness" (premenstrual tension, menstrual headaches). Thus, the
usual treatment of these complaints is to move the blood by treating
certain liver-associated points.

Some of these points are on the Conception Vessel, which runs
through the center of the abdomen and pelvis. One point, "stone gate,"
has the image of a big rusty gate that doesn't open well, which can lead
to liver energy's becoming stuck. Acupuncturists may also choose points
on the foot and leg along the liver channel, in combination with the
spleen, which also governs the blood (detailed in Chapter 7). Sometimes, an acupuncturist uses moxibustion along with the needles, which

warms the acupuncture point, encouraging movement by adding heat.

Although Chinese medicine targets the energy cause and presentation (pain from stuck blood) rather than the Western-defined physiological cause (usually a hormonal imbalance), the two treatment effects are quite similar. It appears that acupuncture actually affects the ability of the body to produce female hormones and restore a proper menstrual cycle. It may also act as an analgesic, much like aspirin or ibuprofen, to relieve pain and discomfort.

For instance, a study published in a 1987 issue of *Obstetrics and Gynecology* followed forty-three women with menstrual cramps and found that more than 90 percent of those treated with acupuncture on a weekly basis for three months showed improvement, compared with just 36 percent of the group receiving placebo treatment with needles. Moreover, women who underwent acupuncture treatment were able to reduce their need for conventional medication in the form of analgesics by more than 40 percent.

## *Pain Management*

Pain, particularly musculoskeletal pain, is one of the most common, most debilitating, and yet least understood conditions that medicine faces. Pain can affect any part of the body and result from any number of conditions. Here in the West, treatment of pain in any part of the body most often consists of a wide range of medications, from aspirin at the lower end of the spectrum to opiates like morphine at the upper end.

Musculoskeletal pain and migraine are among the most studied conditions in acupuncture treatment research. In fact, 67 percent of all acupuncture studies concern treatment of musculoskeletal conditions, and 12 percent concern treatment of headaches. The results of these studies prompted the National Institutes of Health Scientific Consensus Conference Report of 1997 to list the following pain-related conditions as worthy of considering acupuncture: headaches, low back pain, tennis elbow, carpal tunnel syndrome, and osteoarthritis.

Much of the research on the mechanisms of acupuncture has centered on its effects on nerve and muscle function. Doctors know, for instance, that stimulating an acupoint has direct effects on the spinal nerves, as well as the limbic system and midbrain, where pain is perceived and interpreted. It is also known that acupuncture can mitigate the action of the pain messengers of the body and can release endorphins, natural pain-relieving body chemicals. A 1998 study published in the *Clinical Journal of Pain*, for instance, followed forty-six patients with chronic myofascial neck pain, that is, pain in the muscles and the tissue that covers them. Those who underwent acupuncture treatments experienced significantly less pain than did the control groups, which received either sham acupuncture treatments or no treatment at all.

When treating acute pain, acupuncturists usually choose a point at or near the site of the pain to first disperse the inflammation. They may also choose points along the relevant meridians in order to alleviate the deeper problems of blockage and disruption of the flow of *qi* through the channels. Sometimes, an acupuncturist will use a microsystem, such as ear acupuncture or the Yamamoto New Scalp Acupuncture (see Chapter 4), as well as superficial channels called tendinomuscular meridians. Some acupuncturists treat pain by needling acupuncture points that correspond to the nerves connected to the inflamed tissue. The treatment of chronic pain is more complex, usually involving both local and distal points, with a variety of effects.

Musculoskeletal pain (particularly joint pain) is given a special name in Chinese medicine: *bi* syndrome. *Bi* syndrome refers to the obstruction of *qi* and blood in the tissues, mostly due to heat, cold, damp, or other climatic factors that invade the muscles and joints. Many of the musculoskeletal treatments address the removal of the climatic factor, and treat the *bi* syndrome and the organs it affects, such as the liver and spleen. Acupuncturists may also treat musculoskeletal pain with herbs.

Which herbal formula is used depends on whether there is cold, damp, or excess heat (inflammation) in the muscles. The appropriate formulas usually combine "movement" herbs that disperse *qi* with herbs to cool down or heat up the channels, depending on the presentation of symptoms.

As for migraine, most migraine headaches involve an abnormal constriction and dilation of blood vessels in the head, along with other neurological and hormonal factors. Certain environmental or physical factors may act as triggers as well, including certain foods, exposure to allergens such as dander, and muscle tension.

Although migraines can result from various imbalances within the Chinese medical paradigm, the most likely source is a blocked liver energy that causes heat to rise to the head. Acupuncturists treat migraine by stimulating points on the head and lower limbs to soften and reduce the energy. Needling points on the stomach as well as the pericardium point on the wrist helps treat the symptoms of nausea and vomiting often associated with migraine. A randomized, well-controlled trial published in a 1989 issue of the *Clinical Journal of Pain* compared the effects of true and sham acupuncture on thirty patients suffering from chronic migraine. True acupuncture was significantly more effective than the control procedure in reducing pain. The study established that those who underwent true acupuncture experienced a 43 percent reduction in pain and were able to reduce their medication by 38 percent over baseline, as compared to a "sham" treatment: results that were maintained at four-month and one-year follow-up examinations.

Although much more research and controlled testing remains to be done, it seems clear that acupuncture can play a meaningful role in the treatment of pain, which continues to be a stubborn problem for physicians and a debilitating reality for millions of Americans.

## Strengthening Wood Energy with Acupuncture

An imbalance of wood energy may bring on a variety of physical and psychological problems. When treating these symptoms, an acupuncturist will attempt to restore proper balance and flow of *qi* throughout the meridians. As discussed, the underlying cause of the wood energy problem may exist anywhere in the body; a disruption of water energy, for instance, can unbalance wood energy and cause a migraine. However, if the acupuncturist traces the problem to somewhere in the wood element channel or its organs, the treatment will usually include needling one or more of the following points:

• *Liver 3 ("supreme rushing")* Found at the junction of the great toe and second toe, this point is most associated with breaking up blockages and obstructions in the liver channel and elsewhere. It is a source point of the liver channel and is sometimes called "happy calm" for the relaxed, satisfied feeling that can result from a pacified wood energy.

• *Liver 14 ("gate of hope")* Acupuncturists use the last point on the liver meridian, the "gate of hope," to engender in patients a feeling of confidence in the future. Needling this point can help unblock stuck energy, particularly that associated with pain in the chest and abdominal areas. It is located at the bottom of the ribs, below the breast.

• *Gallbladder 41 ("foot above tears")* This point, located on the upper outer surface of the foot, is the horary point. One point in each meridian is a horary point, which means it is particularly active in the season associated with that element, and at specific times of the day. Gallbladder 41 is particularly active from 11 P.M. to 1 A.M., when energy in the gallbladder channel is most active. Acupuncturists use it to treat a broad variety of musculoskeletal pain and other pain syndromes. It is also the exit point on that meridian and thus enables energy that is stuck in the channel to exit.

• *Gallbladder 20 ("wind pond")* As the descriptive name implies, wind enters the body at this point located at the base of the skull, in the notch between the two large neck muscles. When wind enters the body, it can trigger colds and other infections, and thus acupuncturists often use it to treat these conditions. In addition, this point allows energy to leave the head portion of the gallbladder channel, which makes it useful in treating any neck pain, headache, or other head problem.

• *Governing Vessel 20 ("one hundred meetings")* Although not technically a wood point, this point located on the top of the skull, in the midline, is the closest to the heavens of any point and thus is a focal point for *yang* energy. The "meetings" refer to gathering of the wood channels with *yang* channels of the body generally. Needling this point will help alleviate headache and other pain as well as stimulate mental clarity. Acupuncturists may also use it to calm people who have become extremely agitated.

## Maintaining Healthy Wood Energy

The spirit of wood energy is about hope. When one has a clear vision of the future, knows where one is going and how to get there, there is hope. But when all avenues are thwarted and there is no clear pathway, one feels hopeless and frustrated. If you have wood energy and live in balance and health, there is little that can stop you from reaching your goals—or, at least, that can thwart your energy and perseverance. To stay as healthy and vital as possible, adhere to your acupuncturist's treatment plan as well as the following general guidelines:

• *Get moving!* Exercise is the best medicine for wood energy imbalances, which cause muscular tension and emotional stress. Walking is one of the best exercises for wood types, since the visual stimuli involved in taking a stroll may also trigger creativity. Many writers have been known to get new inspiration by going out for a run or a brisk walk. Exercises that stretch and soften muscles, such as yoga and *tai chi*, help relieve pressure and circulate energy throughout the body, which in turn helps to prevent muscle spasms and other injuries. Considering that you have boundless energy when you're feeling healthy, you may even want to take up tennis or mountain biking. Before you do, however, make sure that you're in top form; otherwise, you risk spraining an ankle or suffering from muscle aches and pains.

• *Practice* **qi gong** Here's a *qi gong* movement for activating wood energy: Stand with your feet shoulder-length apart, your knees and elbows bent, and palms facing forward in front of your chest. Since the natural movement of wood is to push forward, up, and out, slowly straighten your legs, and push your palms forward and out. Look ahead toward the horizon, and quietly say "choo" as you move your hands forward. Repeat this movement for several minutes per day.

• *Avoid fatty fast foods* Because of their tendency to rush through life, wood energy types are more apt than other people to depend on convenience foods, which often contain fatty substances that could overburden the liver as well as raise the blood pressure. If you're in this category, instead of eating cheeseburgers and doughnuts, increase your intake of raw, whole foods. Vegetables and fruits will help cleanse your system and provide your body with the vitamins, minerals, and other nutrients it requires to maintain health.

• *Learn to release your anger* Within the Chinese paradigm of health, anger is not a "bad" emotion, unless it is left to fester and disrupt the body as a whole. Regular exercise will help release stress, but so will all of the old standbys: hitting a pillow, closeting yourself in a private place and just yelling out loud, and keeping a journal in which you can express all of your annoyances and frustrations in a safe place.

• *Try some herbal remedies* Many Chinese herbal remedies help to maintain strong wood energy. Those that treat pelvic complaints do so by moving the blood and *qi* of the liver. The free and easy wanderer (*xiao yao wan*), a common Chinese herbal formula, helps to soften and encourage movement of liver energy. Another liver-associated formula, minor bupleurum compound, has been shown in Western studies to reduce hepatitis B (a virus that attacks the liver) viral counts. Angelica sinensis (*dong kuei*) is another herb frequently found in women's herbal formulas. This herb is said to "soften the edge of the liver energy" and to strengthen the blood, encouraging the smooth movement associated with healthy wood. Other common herbs are also used in wood formulas: Dandelion helps to brighten the eyes and to aid vision; licorice helps to harmonize the digestive functions; mint and gentian can help to temper the liver's tendency to heat up into anger and stagnation.

6

# FIRE
## The Spirit Gate

IN THE HEART OF SUMMER, everything is in full bloom. This lushness reflects the vigor of fire energy, bathing the earth in warmth and beauty. Fueled by the heat and light of the sun, plants of all kinds grow tall and luxuriant. We take comfort in the warming touch of the sun's rays as they blanket us, opening to them just like the flowers.

When fire energy is too intense, however, nature becomes scorched and brittle. The heat becomes oppressive, seeming to suck the life from plants, animals, and people. There is drought and damage to crops, threatening food supplies. When fire energy is weak, nature becomes lethargic and sluggish. Without heat to draw them upward from the soil, plants wither and wilt. We feel chilled and uncomfortable, retreating indoors and within ourselves.

## Fire Energy in Health and Disease

If you have fire energy in balance, you are enthusiastic and passionate. You find joy all around you, and you spread joy to others through your infectious and generous laughter. Fire energy longs to be recognized, to be the center of attention. Even in health, there is a desire for connection and recognition. Conversely, someone whose fire energy is in excess can make those around him or her uncomfortable. This person might be the life of the party, but continues to tell jokes and dominate the situation when it's no longer appropriate. The laughter might be too loud, too long. If instead you have fire energy out of balance or in deficit, you might feel morose and uninspired, trudging through each day just because the day forces you to do so.

## The Heart as Emperor

The origins of Chinese medicine come not only from an understanding of the natural universe but also from observations of the proper governance of the empire. In ancient China, the emperor was considered to be a deity. Hidden behind walls of a palace on which few people could ever lay eyes, he had little contact with the outside world of his subjects. Even the courtiers were not privy to the imperial audience except on rare occasions. The emperor had divine power, but the power was in his being, not his actions. That is, the emperor represented perfection and right living, without which there would be chaos. And yet (or perhaps because of this), there was a stability to the vast Chinese empire that lasted for centuries. In many other nations throughout history as well, the role of royalty was simply to "be," to embody the central connectedness of the nation's people, and to symbolize their nearness to the heavens.

In the body, this is the role of the heart, the chief organ of the fire element. In Chinese medicine, the heart is said to be the "emperor," guiding and facilitating the various functions of the other organs and elements. The twelve channels (representing ten organs and two functions, triple heater and pericardium) can be considered officials in that government. Thus, many systems of acupuncture treat the heart sparingly, if at all, preferring to address the emperor through the rest of the court.

Twenty-four centuries ago, Lao-tzu wrote the *Tao-te-ching*, known to us now as *The Tao*, describing a philosophical system in which non-action becomes a powerful force and the motivator for great changes. This concept of action through nonaction is called *wu wei*. As the emperor, the heart governs through the principle of *wu wei*, that is, governing through nonaction. In terms of acupuncture, this means that the heart is not often treated directly, but its influences are evident in the treatment of the rest of the fire energy, along with the other organs.

## The Emperor's Ministers

Just as the emperor needs a close minister who filters everything so that the emperor will receive only what is pure, the heart has such an organ: the small intestine. Termed the "sorter of the pure from the impure," it is the *yang* organ paired with the *yin* heart organ. The small intestine acts as a filter, ensuring that only the purest of food, energy, emotions, and spirit reaches the heart.

Unique to the fire energy are two other aspects, not organs in the physical sense, but rather serving more as functional organs. They are considered separate parts of the fire element and are paired. The *yin* organ is the pericardium, or "heart protector" in Five-Element terminology. Other names include "master of the heart" (French energetics) and "circulation-sex." The pericardium acts as the guard at the door to the inner chamber of the heart, allowing entry and exit in appropriate situations. The *yang* functional organ is called the triple heater (triple energizer in international terminology). It takes the message from the emperor and distributes it to the population. Thus, the triple heater is responsible for harmonizing the entire empire of the body, mind, and spirit, making sure all aspects are on the same page.

The heart is also called the "supreme controller." Its pathway, the upper *shao yin* (see Figure 2), begins in the armpit, where it connects deeply to the heart. It then descends the ulnar side of the arm and forearm, ending at the pinky. There, it connects to the small intestine, or upper *tai yang*, pathway. This pathway ascends from the pinky and runs up the ulnar side of the arm to the back of the armpit, where it zigzags across the shoulder-blade area, up the side of the neck, and onto the jaw. It ends in the angle of the jaw in front of the ear, at a point called the "listening palace."

The pericardium channel, also called upper *jue yin*, begins at the side of the pectoral muscle, lateral to the breast (see Figure 2). It goes around the front of the shoulder and down the center of the arm and forearm, ending on the middle finger. The triple heater, or upper *shao yang*, begins on the fourth finger and goes up the outside of the arm, over the elbow and side of the shoulder, and then up the neck, behind the ear (see Figure 3). After looping behind the ear, it ends on the temple, where it sends a connection to its *shao yang* partner, the gallbladder. Along the way, the triple heater sends branches to each of the three body spaces (chest, abdomen, and pelvis), thus giving the channel its name.

## Fire Energy in Balance

Fire represents joy and laughter. People with strong fire energy frequently meet the world with jokes, laughter, and a sunny affect. They are warm, loving, and welcoming in their nature. Their appropriate laughter and joy signal that the element is in balance. In addition, the "heart protector" gives the fire element an aspect of intimacy. Healthy intimacy means being able to feel vulnerable and yet not lose yourself in the vulnerability to the extent that your identity is attacked. In a sense, it means that the "heart protector" guards the chambers of the heart, letting in warmth and love, and keeping out anything that is dangerous or threatening. Finally, the triple heater gives a great sense of balance and harmony to the healthy fire energy, allowing each of the organs to perform its functions in concert with the others.

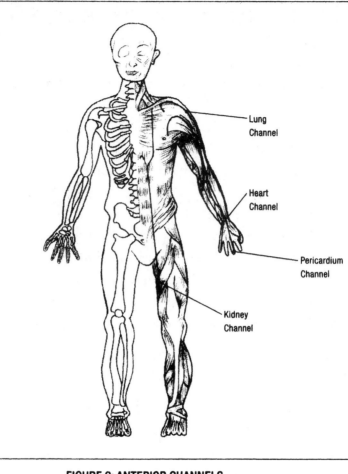

**FIGURE 2: ANTERIOR CHANNELS**

Think of a burning fire. A strong fire burns steadily, warming every-one and everything around it. It needs to be stoked from time to time but not constantly. It is unpredictable, with each moment offering a new look, but at the same time reassuring in its light and heat. This describes someone who has healthy fire energy.

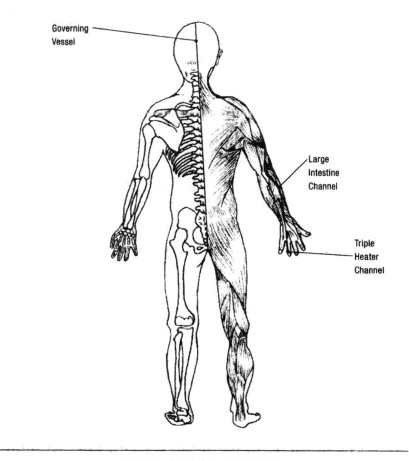

**FIGURE 3: POSTERIOR CHANNELS**

# Fire Energy Out of Balance

As explained at the beginning of the chapter, sometimes the fire element is out of balance. As is true for the other elements, this condition can result in excess or deficiency.

In diagnosing excess fire, a practitioner considers the appropriateness of the situation. For instance, I have a patient who always greets me with a boisterous "How are ya, Doc?" and answers my question about his chronic back pain by exploding in laughter and stating, "Lousy as ever." However pleasant this man is to be with, his joy and laughter are out of sync with the fact that he's in constant, disabling pain.

Deficient fire energy is more common. Every day, medical practitioners see patients who describe feeling flat and having no joy in their lives. These people present their stories in monotones, without spontaneous joy or humor. When we interact with them in a humorous way, they might brighten up for a moment; they are responding to the fire energy of others. However, after the moment is gone, they are back to their flat affect.

In most people with fire energy imbalance, the pericardium/circulation-sex has been affected. That is, in some formative situation or situations in their lives, their intimacy was breached by something that felt unsafe. This experience could range from growing up in a family with weak or nonexistent boundaries and thus filled with interactions that felt invasive, to an actual rape or other abusive event. It is as if the door to the emperor's inner chamber has been broken from its hinges. It can be repaired, but it may not fit quite as snugly as before.

After such an event and the feelings it engenders, a person becomes always a bit guarded, especially in new situations or situations with potential intimacy. Energy circulates in the chest, guarding the heart, but does not circulate as easily into the rest of the body. Thus, the person may develop symptoms in the arms and legs, such as carpal tunnel syndrome or Raynaud's syndrome, a condition in which the hands and feet become extremely cold. Muscles and tissues tighten to help protect the heart. The result can be muscular chest pain, tightness in the neck and upper back, and shallow breathing. The immune system and the fight-or-flight response, two systems that guard the body from "invaders," become hyperactive, leading to allergies and autoimmune disease. Laughter and joking can be absent, or they can be tools to avoid closer interactions. Depression can follow.

## Fire Energy and the Spirit

The fire element, then, is all about the heart and what it symbolizes. And one need only look to the great literature of the world to see what the heart symbolizes. *Love, passion,* and *spirited joy* are all words associated with the heart. In English, we have the concept of a "broken heart" to describe someone who is deeply saddened when the bonds that draw a partner or loved one close are severed. "A merry heart maketh a cheerful countenance: but by sorrow of the heart the spirit is broken," is written in the Bible (Proverbs, 15:13). Likewise, in Chinese medicine, the emotion of the fire energy is joy, and its vocal sound is laughter.

Critical to the joy that is the fire element and held in the heart is the concept that the heart is the residence of the *shen*, or spirit. All of the elements include spiritual aspects, but the *shen* is closest to what we think of as spirit. In health, the *shen* is lively, strong, and vibrant. In Chinese medicine, a healthy *shen* is likened to the spirit of a wild horse. The eyes are clear and able to hold a gaze. The mind is open and relaxed. The body is strong and supple. There is hope, energy, and a connection to the possibilities of the surrounding world.

There isn't an easy way of expressing the spiritual realm in medical terms. Chinese medicine deals with the body, mind, and spirit in terms that are equally descriptive, specific, and concrete. When the *shen* is weakened, the eyes are dull. The body can sag or can be tense and in constant movement. The mind is agitated, sometimes not staying on one topic for any length of time. There is restlessness and sometimes even psychosis or disordered thinking.

Many points in acupuncture address the spirit; most of these are on the front or back of the chest, in the vicinity of the heart. "Spirit bur-

ial ground," "spirit hall," and "spirit storehouse" are names of points on
the chest that lie on either the kidney or bladder channel. Other points,
such as "utmost source" and "spirit gate," are located on the heart channel directly. Needling "one hundred meetings" helps bring mental calm,
as does needling *shen men* (a point on the ear). Acupuncturists use these
points to address depression and mental agitation.

## The Inner Frontier Gate: Acupuncture and the Immune System

The body has several systems that protect it from the outside world. The
skin, for instance, protects the entire body from easy invasion by environmental hazards, and the fight-or-flight response gets the heart
pumping and the muscles warm in case you need to either run from danger or stand and fight it.

Perhaps the largest area of protection is the immune system. It lines
the digestive and respiratory tracts, and makes up a portion of the blood
and lymph systems. Comprising antibodies and blood cells, which protect the body from invasion by infections and foreign substances, the
immune system can overreact, responding to agents such as dust or mold
in ways that are out of proportion to their threat. This is called allergy.
In my practice, I see many patients with allergies to foods, to inhalants,
and to chemicals in the environment. Some of these patients are allergic enough to be called environmentally sensitive, and they can be quite
disabled by their allergic symptoms. I see a common pattern in many of
these patients, related to weakness of the "heart protector."

As an example, one of my patients is a middle-aged woman who has
become progressively more sensitive to the world around her. She is
unable to be in carpeted rooms due to the fumes that she can smell. Even
coming to the office can feel like an obstacle course to her, for fear of
exposure to noxious odors. Her diet consists of very few foods, since
most foods give her dizziness, weakness, numbness and tingling, and

even a dulling of her thought processes. She has a history of incest in childhood and has undergone much therapy to heal the effects. She has spent much of her adult life mildly depressed and alone.

This is an extreme example, but this woman's fire energy, particularly her "heart protector," was injured early in her life, resulting in an enhanced vulnerability in her adulthood. In effect, she does not feel safe in the world around her, and her body has become hypervigilant to any possible danger, no matter how benign it really is. Her immune system and her fight-or-flight response are hyperreactive. Although such traumas can affect every aspect of one's energy, the "heart protector" is particularly impacted, with immune hyperreactivity the result. Treatment of this condition is complex, but I have found acupuncture to be helpful in many cases. It can help to needle the "inner frontier gate," an important point on the pericardium channel whose name implies the protection of intimacy that is so critical to the fire element.

## Treating Fire Energy Imbalance

When I walk into the room to see a new patient, I usually find the person seated next to the desk, where it's obvious I will be conducting the first part of the interview. Occasionally, however, a patient will be seated in the chair on the far side of the room, away from the desk and me. He or she will greet me warily. Sometimes, the person will warm up to my attempts at humor and friendliness; in other cases, the person will maintain the guardedness. On exam, I typically will find tight upper back and neck muscles and tenderness along the breastbone, signs of a lot of energy concentrated around the chest. The hands and feet will be cold, sometimes with tenderness over the carpal tunnel of the wrist or on areas of the arms and legs. Pupils will be wide, the skin sensitive to touch and sometimes clammy. The lower *chou* (below the umbilicus) will feel cooler, as though energy does not travel down that far. Allergies, or even chemical sensitivities, are commonly reported, as are palpitations and anxiety. The pulse feels weak and thready in the third position, where the fire pulses are found.

When I am confronted with this situation, I almost always know that some trauma, either specific or general, has occurred. As an acupuncturist, I don't need to know the details or even whether the patient is aware of it, although sometimes it is helpful to articulate for patients what they already know inside. Rather, I need to know that the "heart protector"/heart energy has been wounded, leaving the patient feeling vulnerable, hypervigilant, and unable to experience unbridled joy. In my practice, this is the root of many chronic environmental-sensitivity syndromes. It is also the source of many chronic low-level depression and anxiety syndromes that I see commonly, and I address them by treating the fire energy and its supporting organs.

The symptoms of depression, particularly with anxiety, can mimic those of heart problems, with patients reporting palpitations, shortness of breath, and chest pains. This reflects the heart's connection to the fire energy. Being depressed, in turn, drains heart energy. Of course, anyone with these symptoms should consult a medical doctor. Once the cause has been determined, Chinese medicine can be utilized to restore energy balance.

Western medicine often employs treatments consisting of counseling, psychotherapy, or drugs, sometimes in combination. A parallel, albeit a limited one, exists between Western medicine's use of therapy in which the patient talks about his or her problems in an attempt to identify and resolve them and Chinese medicine. Heart energy has to do with communication, and thus, there is a connection of the heart channel to the tongue and correspondingly between emotions and talking.

In Chinese medicine, some point combinations can be used to treat depression and "spirit-level" problems. One popular treatment involves a series of points called "releasing the dragons." The "dragons" are actually helpful in controlling chaotic aspects of the mind and spirit. Insomnia is often a symptom of depression, frequently due to a "restless *shen*," and can be treated by using the heart and associated channels, along with some of the points that address the spirit.

The climate factor associated with fire is, of course, heat. Sometimes, our internal thermometers get out of balance, leading to hot and cold sensations that are out of proportion to environmental conditions. Treatment of the triple heater can frequently resolve such excess heat or cold sensations in the body, or even in parts of the body, such as heat sensations in the head, or feelings of cold in the lower body.

Many musculoskeletal conditions are addressed through fire meridian treatments. The small intestine channel (see Figure 4 and Figure 6) covers the back of the shoulder and side of the neck. Frequently, tension in this area impedes circulation and energy in the upper limb, preventing arm and hand problems such as carpal tunnel syndrome from healing. The carpal tunnel itself, a tendon covering on the wrist, is right over an area of the pericardium channel, where it is usually treated with acupuncture. Also, pain in the armpit area can involve the heart channel, which originates here.

Drug and alcohol dependency is another area in which acupuncture has been demonstrated to be useful. While it is impossible to attribute such a complex problem to a single aspect of energy, it is the job of the small intestine to provide the heart with pure substances. Thus, the small intestine is found to be imbalanced in many cases of drug addiction, and treating this site, along with the heart and other channels, can lead to better choices for the body, mind, and spirit.

When you visit an acupuncturist and your fire energy is imbalanced, the practitioner will develop a treatment plan that includes one or more therapies from the Eightfold Path. Some of the specific acupoints used to strengthen fire energy are listed later in the chapter. In addition to needling those points, your acupuncturist may decide to treat your symptoms with herbal medicine or exercise and—considering the importance of mental calm and well-being—may suggest that you learn to meditate.

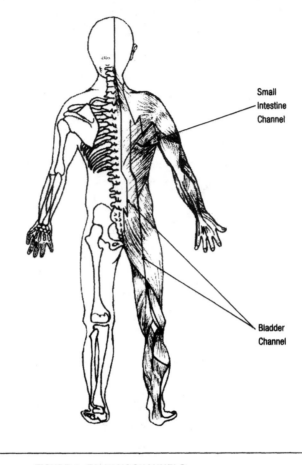

Small
Intestine
Channel

Bladder
Channel

**FIGURE 4: *TAI YANG* CHANNELS**

## *Meditation: To Quiet the Spirit*

Meditation is a mental exercise that affects body processes. People all over the world, in every culture and on every continent, practice meditation. It is effective both in reducing general stress and in helping to relax a body and mind made tense by anxiety or worry. When you meditate, you quiet your nervous system, thereby reducing the state of muscle contraction. Meditation can help you psychologically by allowing you to focus on the cause of your stress and find ways to change the way you respond to the challenges you face. Researchers have found that people who meditate regularly tend to come away with more positive feelings after a stressful encounter, sleep better, and tackle challenges with more confidence.

Within the Chinese tradition, meditation is another therapeutic means of nurturing and balancing the human energy system. When you meditate, you draw healing energy into your system from nature and the cosmos. This involves freeing the mind from all external stimuli and finding a concentrated mental and emotional quiet and a sustained physical relaxation. Some methods of meditation use the breath and steady, focused breathing to concentrate energy.

Meditation for relaxation can be done at any time of the day and in any comfortable space. All it takes is about fifteen minutes in a quiet place where you can remain undisturbed. One easy, more Western way to meditate incorporates the relaxation response, invented in the 1970s by Dr. Herbert Benson, as cited earlier. The relaxation response works to bring a stressed body and mind back into balance quickly and efficiently. The following deep-breathing exercise may help you trigger this relaxation response whenever you begin to feel overstressed:

1. Sit on the floor in a comfortable position, with your back straight and your head erect.
2. Close your eyes and concentrate only on your breathing. Leave behind the worries of the day and think only of this moment of time. Feel your breath as it flows into your mouth and nose and down into your lungs.
3. As you breathe in, picture your body filling with energy, light, and air. Feel your chest and upper back open up as air enters the body. The inhalation should take about five seconds.
4. When your lungs feel comfortably full, stop the movement and the intake of air. Exhale in a controlled, smooth, continuous movement, with the air streaming steadily out of your nostrils.

5. Repeat the inhalation-exhalation about four times a minute, resting two or three seconds between breaths, until you feel relaxed.

6. If you like, add a self-affirmation to your meditation session by saying something positive to yourself every time you exhale, such as, "I am in control. I am relaxed. I am able to manage my life."

Chinese medicine has its own form of standing meditation. It serves as the basic beginning posture of *qi gong* and can be used by itself to clear the mind, calm the spirit, and build energy in the lower belly, or *dan tien*, the seat of energy.

The exercise is performed standing, with the feet shoulder-length apart and the knees slightly bent. Imagine that a point on the top of your head is being pulled up toward the sky and that, at the same time, a point on the soles of your feet is connected to the earth. Bend your arms and hold an imaginary ball of energy at waist height. The ball can be small or large, depending on the distance from one another at which your palms feel most comfortable. Concentrate on the ball of *qi*, letting all other thoughts drift in and out. Breathe slowly and deeply, and let your eyes soften without focusing on anything.

Hold this posture for five to ten minutes, allowing all thoughts to drift away. When you catch yourself thinking of something specific, bring your attention back to the ball of energy in front of your belly. When you are done, place your hands on your lower belly for a few minutes, and then "wash" your face with your hands. Doing this simple exercise every day will have remarkable restorative effects on your body, mind, and spirit.

## Treating Depression and Anxiety

Chemical depression results from an imbalance of neurotransmitters in the brain, such as serotonin and dopamine. These substances work in the nervous system to create states of relaxation, well-being, and spontaneity. When the neurotransmitters are depleted, depression occurs. The most common medications used to treat depression are called selective serotonin reuptake inhibitors (SSRIs) because they prevent serotonin from being eliminated from the brain.

In Chinese medicine, depression can result from an imbalance of any element, but ultimately, fire energy and the heart are affected, since the heart is the seat of the *shen*. Thus, most acupuncture treatments geared toward treating depression, anxiety, or even sleep disturbances will include some fire points. The *shen* is said to be restless and in need of soothing.

Two randomized controlled trials have compared the effects of electroacupuncture and amitriptyline hydrochloride (a commonly prescribed antidepressant) in 270 depressed patients. By using a standardized scale to assess the level of the illness, researchers determined that both groups scored equally well in experiencing relief from the depression. Acupuncture had significantly better effects than the drug in some symptoms such as disturbance of thought processes and anxiety, and the chance of this finding being coincidental was less than 5 percent (in statistical terms, this is written $P < 0.05$). Furthermore, after two to four years, the recurrence rates for depression were equal in both groups, meaning that the acupuncture group had effects as lasting as the group taking antidepressants.

In another study of chronically ill patients (*Journal of Acupuncture*, 1986), this one uncontrolled, a physician measured the fluctuation in levels of anxiety and depression before and after one month of acupuncture treatments. Forty-two out of sixty anxiety patients and forty-five out of fifty depressed patients returned to normal after they were given acupuncture treatments.

Acupuncture probably aids depression and anxiety by its activity on the brain neurotransmitters. In rabbits, acupuncture raises brain levels of 5-hydroxytryptophan, which is the precursor for serotonin. In other animal studies, electroacupuncture was shown to increase the production of both serotonin and another neurotransmitter, norepinephrine, in the central nervous system.

## *Treating Addiction*

Addiction research has burgeoned as this societal problem has become more visible. Because results of other approaches have been mixed, interest has grown in the use of acupuncture for substance withdrawal. As a result, more than 5 percent of the world literature on acupuncture pertains to its use in addiction treatment. While studies of using acupuncture to aid withdrawal have included alcohol, cigarettes, prescription drugs, cocaine, and even overeating, most of the literature pertains to its use with heroin addiction and other opiates.

The landmark study of acupuncture's success in treating addiction took place in the early 1970s, when researchers at Hong Kong's Kwa Wah Hospital used electroacupuncture (see Chapter 4) to treat thirty opium and ten heroin addicts (Wen & Cheung, 1973). The study's participants experienced measurable relief from the symptoms of withdrawal and ultimately became free from addiction (with the exception of one person who dropped out of the study). Though not considered definitive by today's standards, the study nonetheless established the groundwork for using electroacupuncture. In the late 1970s, researchers at the University of Hawaii tried electroacupuncture and achieved similar results. These researchers also established that electroacupuncture was most effective in people with mild to moderate addictions and who had no other medical problems. Subsequent studies over the next two decades, conducted in various settings, affirmed acupuncture's effectiveness as a treatment for addiction.

Also in the 1970s, Dr. Michael Smith began using and studying acupuncture in treating addiction at New York City's Lincoln Hospital. By the mid-1980s, the program was treating two hundred addicts a day. In 1985, Smith was appointed director of the National Acupuncture Detoxification Association (NADA), an organization established to train acupuncturists in treating addiction. In 1988 in the *Bulletin on Narcotics*, he summarized the program's approach to using acupuncture to relieve the symptoms of withdrawal and help people to stay drug-free. One element of the Lincoln Hospital program that differed from other studies was the integration of acupuncture with other treatment methods, including group therapy, individual counseling, and services to address the many social issues of addiction.

Ear acupuncture points for the sympathetic nervous system, *shen men* (a commonly used point that accompanies many ear treatments), lung, kidney, and liver are most commonly used, though the acupuncturist always determines which points to target based on the person's unique circumstances and needs. Studies of the use of acupuncture to treat addiction to nicotine (which is as addictive as opiates) are more limited, but they produce similar findings. Many people also experience acupuncture, particularly electroacupuncture, to be useful in managing alcohol withdrawal as well as in staying free from alcohol use.

Another area in which acupuncture shows great promise is in treating addiction to benzodiazepines (the family of drugs to which Valium, Librium, and Atavan, among others, belong). The most commonly prescribed drugs to treat a wide range of psychiatric conditions, benzodiazepines are addictive even when taken therapeutically (i.e., as prescribed). As many as half the people who take them will end up addicted.

Acupuncture, and again particularly electroacupuncture, seems to provide the same kind of relief from the symptoms of withdrawal as it does for withdrawal from opiates and nicotine. However, there are few clinical studies to corroborate this perception.

### Boosting Immunity

Acupuncture affects the body's immune system both in ways that are understood and in ways that remain unclear. Practitioners of acupuncture view immunity as multifactorial, meaning that it has many dimensions and influences beyond what Western medicine defines as the immune system. Some of the most exciting research taking place is in the area of psychoneuroimmunology—a blend of the mind (psycho), the brain and nervous system (neuro), and the immune system. In the lab, researchers use experiments that relate an action and an expectation in order to produce an outcome. One example is a study in which lab animals received a drug to suppress their immune systems, along with a strongly flavored drink. After repeating this a number of times, researchers were able to give the animals the drink alone and measure a response in the immune system similar to what was observed with the drug (decreases in certain kinds of cells in the blood).

The practical application of these studies for people has to do with the relationship between stress, particularly grief, and the ability to ward off illness and disease. Doctors have observed for centuries that people are unusually susceptible to illness when they are grieving. Until the twentieth century, however, the technology did not exist to examine and measure this connection. Researchers now know that certain intense emotional states lower the number of certain immune-system cells, and other components of the immune system.

Acupuncture can offset this depression, both by affecting its process and by restoring balance to the emotional state. One controlled study (*Journal of Traditional Chinese Medicine*, 1988) showed an increase in phagocytic activity (the cleanup function of immune cells) in acupuncture patients, compared with controls. Though other studies have shown a response to acupuncture in various immune cells, information in this area is far from complete or definitive; there is much still to be learned. Nevertheless, the prospects are quite promising.

❖

### *Restoring Fire Energy Balance with Acupuncture*

The following are the acupuncture points that are most often used to treat fire energy imbalances:

• *Heart 7 ("spirit gate")* The source, or *yuan* point, of the heart channel is used to address the essence of the heart. It is on the inside ulnar surface of the wrist.

• *Pericardium 6 ("inner frontier gate")* Found on the inside surface of the arm centrally near the wrist, this is one of the most utilized points on the body. It is a junction point and connects with the triple heater. It is useful in calming the spirit, in treating nausea and vomiting, and as part of a Five-Element treatment to address the vulnerability associated with the "heart protector."

• *Triple heater 4 ("harmony bone")* As its descriptive name implies, this source point captures the energy of the triple heater, which harmonizes the various areas of the body that it traverses. The point is on the back of the wrist and can be used in conjunction with other treatments to bring balance and equanimity.

• *Small intestine 19 ("listening palace")* The exit point of the small intestine channel, this point is one that acupuncturists needle in order to allow stuck energy to move from this channel into the bladder meridian. It is in the angle of the jaw, in front of the ear, and is useful in treating problems of the jaw as well as hearing difficulties.

# Keeping the Fire Burning: Maintaining a Healthy Balance

Having your fire energy out of balance can be intensely uncomfortable for you as well as for others around you. If your fire energy is depleted, you feel depressed and out of sorts—not someone others want to be around (and you might not even want to be around yourself!). If you are hypersensitive, hostile, and angry, you won't be able to recharge and reenergize yourself. Here are some ways to help restore and maintain the balance of your fire energy:

• *Bring joy into your life* Make an effort to see all the good that is around you and to take part in activities that are fun.

• *Get enough sleep* Sleep recharges you; in combination with a nutritious diet and plenty of exercise, it gives you the resources to handle the challenges that life throws at you.

• *Stay away from addictive substances* Alcohol, drugs, and cigarettes are problems, not solutions. They create imbalance, not just in your fire energy but in all dimensions of your life.

• *Follow a path of right living* Within the Eightfold Path Toward Health, this path is both the purest and most difficult. Thousands of years ago, it was recognized that a life filled with wisdom, charity, and moderate behavior leads to a healthy spirit, a clear mind, and a strong body. These principles underlie most civilized cultures and support the concept of living with "a pure heart."

• *Bolster your energy with Chinese herbs* Several formulas in Chinese medicine address the spirit aspect of the fire energy. They are usually used for the symptoms of insomnia and depression. A common formula called *an mian pian* (which means "restless sleep pill") is used to help anxiety and insomnia. Jujube, zizyphus, and biota seeds are common single herbs added to formulas to address restless *shen* problems such as anxiety, depression, and insomnia. Cinnamon twig combination, a formula used to treat emotional vulnerability, is traditionally used to strengthen the immune system, but it can be used as well to address the inability to ward off emotional trauma, as with someone who is easily embarrassed or unable to open up to intimate relationships.

• *Try qi gong for balance* To soothe and warm the heart, try this exercise: While standing, hold your left arm outward to the side. With your right palm on your chest, massage your heart by rubbing the area around the breast in a circular motion. Softly repeat the word "ho." This should be performed for several minutes per day.

# 7

# EARTH
## Abundant Splendor

EARTH ENERGY IS THE ENERGY of the late summer, when the fruits of human labor and the creative spirit yield the bounty of the soil. Earth energy is the mothering energy, the energy that grounds us and nurtures us. The earth gives us our food. When the earth is moist and rich, it produces a harvest of food rich with flavor, color, and nutrients. When it is parched and compact, it cannot provide the same bounty; the food it bears is dry and spindly. When the earth is too wet, it becomes bogged down and smothers everything within it.

The acts of eating and digestion represent the earth energy's expression in human terms. Eating both satisfies one of our most basic needs and provides one of our most sensual pleasures. We eat for energy, for the nutrients that the cells of the body require. We also eat to comfort ourselves, to quell our anxieties and insecurities. Who has not dealt with stress by reaching for a bag of cookies or a bowl of popcorn? We also eat as a way of extending and deepening personal relationships. We eat together as families, as friends, as business colleagues. The smell of Grandmother's cooking stays with us as a warm and nourishing memory throughout our lives.

If your earth energy is in balance, your nature is caring, compassionate, and, above all, tolerant. You have many friends of different types, and you refrain from judging others. Although you have opinions and hold them passionately, you also embrace diversity. You seek to establish connections with others, and you ask only for one thing in return: honesty.

If you have strong earth energy, you're probably often the one at whose house everyone gathers. You feed them, both physically and emotionally. Food, of course, is an important part of your life and is a means by which you nourish yourself and others. Over meals, you listen to people's problems and offer sympathy and consolation. They appreciate your solid grounding and common sense. You are a good teacher and a wise counselor.

Physically, people with strong earth energy typically struggle with weight at times. Earth is round, and so the face, belly, and even hands and fingers tend to have a roundness to them. Sweets can be their downfall, although they're not apt to gorge. They like to touch and be touched, whether it is a gentle pat on the hand or a back rub.

## Earth Energy in Health and Disease

Considering the nurturing aspect of earth energy, it should come as no surprise that, in terms of human health, earth energy largely involves the digestive system. In fact, most digestive disorders can be traced to an imbalance of earth energy in some way, even if the cause of the imbalance is elsewhere. Some of the most common digestive problems and their treatment from a traditional Chinese medicine perspective are detailed later in the chapter.

Within the Five-Element paradigm, the two organs of the earth element—the stomach and spleen—play central roles in the digestive process. The stomach has the role of rotting and ripening. It processes the nourishment we provide it when we eat—churning the food, mixing it with digestive juices, and making it usable by the body. The natural movement of the stomach energy is downward, through the gut. Thus, movement upward, as in nausea and vomiting, is considered a problem of the movement of stomach *qi*. The spleen has the job of transportation and distribution. Once the stomach breaks down the food we eat and makes it usable, the spleen moves the nutrients through the body, to every cell of every organ and tissue.

Several other organs function within the earth element. The stomach channel (see Figure 5) has points both at the corners of the mouth and on the jaw, involving the muscles of chewing and salivary production. In fact, the mouth itself is a digestive organ, and the production of saliva starts the digestive process, along with the act of chewing. Also, as discussed in Chapter 4, the tongue is used in Chinese medicine as a diagnostic tool, especially to reflect the state of digestion, and it too is part of the earth element.

## Earth Energy Out of Balance

To understand the experience of earth energy imbalance, try to imagine what it feels like to be hungry all the time. There is a Buddhist image, the "hungry ghost," whose mouth is the size of a mosquito and whose stomach is as big as the ocean. The hungry ghost wanders the world, never able to feel satisfied. This is the experience of earth imbalance.

Within the Five-Element paradigm, the climate most related to the earth element is dampness. Outside of the digestive system, dampness is anything that bogs us down. One's house is filled with books not quite read, never-sorted papers, clothes piled in a hamper. Dampness can drag us down and make us feel as if we are walking through molasses. Physically, dampness causes gas and pain in the intestines, as well as fluid in the legs that makes walking difficult. Feeling heavy-headed, as if the thoughts have to move through fog, likewise implies a dampness condition. The dampness can also be localized, as in a wound that is puffy and weeping or an arthritic joint that is swollen and achy when the weather is damp.

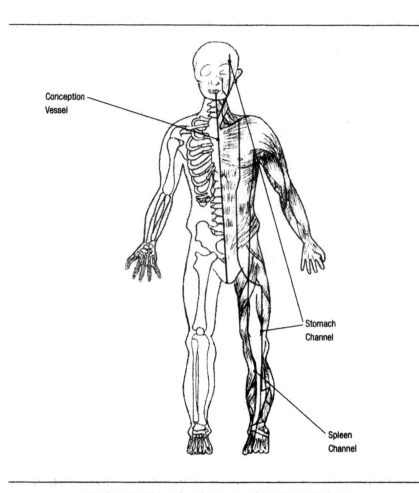

Conception Vessel

Stomach Channel

Spleen Channel

**FIGURE 5: EARTH CHANNELS AND CONCEPTION VESSEL**

## The Earth Motivator

When it comes to the life of the mind and spirit, people with an earth imbalance are always looking for nurturing and never receiving enough. They want to tell others about their problems, and they lavish details on the descriptions of those problems. They respond overtly to sympathy and mothering, usually with excitement that someone "understands" them. Their need for nurturing suggests someone who loves to be waited on, fed, cared for, and babied. One former patient of mine is a classic example. He was forty-seven years old, overweight, and living with his elderly mother, who delighted in feeding him and who accompanied him to every appointment to make sure that I understood how difficult his conditions were to care for. (Clearly, this was a situation of two imbalances—mother's and son's.)

Someone with an earth energy imbalance brings every conversation around to his or her own troubles and cannot move out of a self-focus that can seem very narrow to others. A family acquaintance of mine is a woman with fibromyalgia, and nary a gathering occurs that isn't punctuated with a blow-by-blow description of her latest complication or failed treatment. Another common type is the long-sufferer, someone who denies having any problems but does so in a way that lets everyone know just how bad things are.

In acupuncture school, my colleagues and I used the acronym PLOM, which stood for Poor Li'l Old Me, to describe certain patients. As students, we would watch some patients walk jauntily from the parking lot to the door, appearing to be hale and in good spirits, only to then slowly and painfully limp across the waiting room to the receptionist desk. These patients clearly wanted, on some level, to make sure that we understood just how painful their situations were, even if they could—and often did—feel a little better than they wanted to appear. This behavior, too, is typical of an earth element out of balance.

To understand what happens when the stomach doesn't do its job, as occurs with an earth element imbalance, all you need to do is observe a cow chewing its cud. Cows repeatedly masticate their food, moving it through and between their four stomachs, in order to slowly extract the nutrition from it. In comparison, someone with a stomach imbalance can seem to be endlessly going over the same issue, constantly looking for the answer to his or her problems but never actually able to come to a firm determination about either the problem or its solution.

Of course, these are not conscious behaviors. Nor are they abnormal. All of us have tendencies that form our personalities, and none of us is in perfect balance. Perhaps you see yourself in the description of someone who is never quite satiated, who is always ruminating on something, never seeming to bring anything to fruition. Perhaps you are like the soil that is too damp to hold a good crop, like the fruit that never ripens on the vine, like the land too parched and exhausted to hold the richness and fertility that guarantee a future. If so, Chinese medicine would say that your earth energy needs treatment. In that case, acupuncture and its adjunct treatments can bring the promise of fullness and satisfaction.

## The Earth Granary

When the earth organs cannot transform raw materials into usable energy, dampness occurs. Basically, the intestines are not able to distill the food we eat and to transport it to the appropriate organs and tissues, and the resulting dampness in the intestines can induce belching, sour feeling in the abdomen, diarrhea, bloating, and sticky tongue coating. In addition, gastrointestinal reflux disorder, nausea, and vomiting are symptoms of the stomach energy's moving in the wrong direction, and treatment of this imbalance will help.

Further down in the intestines, the function of the spleen comes into play. Inability to properly digest, absorb, and assimilate indicates an imbalance of the spleen energy. Bloating, gas, and dull aching in the abdomen are signs that the spleen is not functioning well. So-called functional bowel disease (which includes irritable bowel syndrome) usually involves an abnormal condition of the spleen and is treated as such with acupuncture. Other bowel diseases such as Crohn's disease and ulcerative colitis (collectively called inflammatory bowel disease) also indicate a derangement of the spleen energy.

In addition to digestive disturbances, many other conditions can result from earth energy problems. Other organs in the body are involved with nurturing, particularly the breast and uterus, and problems of each are frequently treated with points on earth channels. In fact, the stomach channel runs right through the center of the breast on its way to the digestive organs, and the spleen channel sends a deep branch that penetrates the uterus.

Since the spleen is said to control the flow of blood, it is basic to problems of menstruation, although the cyclical nature of the wood element is critical as well (see Chapter 5).

The pathway of the stomach channel begins at the lower eye, and while visual problems are usually associated with the wood channels, irritation of the eyelids and tearing can be earth problems. Headaches, particularly on the temples where the stomach channels lie, can signify an earth energy imbalance, as can problems of the groin and thighs as the channel moves lower along the body. Finally, pain in the armpits can signify difficulty in the spleen energy's traversing deeper into the body at this point and reexiting at the heart channel.

## Treating Earth Energy Imbalance

If your earth energy is affected and you suffer from the kinds of conditions just cited, your main goal—and the goal of your traditional Chinese medical practitioner—is to bring your earth energy back into balance. The dampness that has resulted from this imbalance has clogged your system, causing you to become bogged down and stuck. In order to feel healthy again, you must work at becoming unstuck, emotionally, physically, and spiritually.

Depending on the specific set of symptoms you present, your practitioner will use a combination of acupuncture, dietary therapy, and other aspects of the Eightfold Path Toward Health as discussed in Chapter 4. This chapter will explain how traditional Chinese medicine, and specifically acupuncturists, treat gastrointestinal reflux disorder, irritable bowel syndrome, and nausea and vomiting. First, however, it's helpful to better understand one of the most important areas of the earth element: diet and nutrition. Perhaps more than any other type in the Five-Element paradigm, a person ruled primarily by the earth energy must first address his or her dietary habits in order to maintain balance and health.

## Harvesting the Earth's Bounty

The perspective of a traditional Chinese practitioner in considering diet and nutrition differs from that of a Western physician. In order to bring you back into balance using dietary therapy, the practitioner carefully evaluates your particular physical makeup and specific symptoms. So, even two people diagnosed with the same earth element imbalance (irritable bowel syndrome, for instance) will require different dietary prescriptions in order to alleviate the symptoms and restore underlying balance. Notwithstanding, some general guidelines apply to earth energy problems.

If your system is dominated by earth energy, chances are you love to eat. Food both nourishes and comforts you, and feeding yourself and others makes you feel complete and satisfied. You probably have a tendency to overeat and—because any imbalance in earth energy may result in digestive problems—have difficulty in controlling your weight. When you're out of balance, you probably head for sweets—cookies, pastries, chocolate—which only creates more problems for you (as is true of the population in general).

If you have trouble controlling your diet and/or suffer from digestive problems related to an earth energy imbalance, an acupuncturist may offer one or more of these recommendations:

• *Add water* Drinking at least eight 8-ounce glasses of water every day will help you in many ways. First, you'll probably eat less, because water tends to fill you up. Second, having plenty of fluid in your system helps move the food through the digestive tract with more ease. Though it's counterintuitive, drinking water can reduce a damp condition by helping to remove toxins.

• *Always cook your foods* Traditional Chinese medical theory holds that eating raw food puts stress on the spleen, which is the organ responsible for breaking down and extracting essential nutrients from food. Thus, soups and stews, for instance, are good spleen-nourishing foods. Many common Chinese meals, such as chow mein, are mixtures of vegetables, meat, and sauce. You cook the ingredients until they are soft, which helps nurture the spleen.

• *Avoid fatty foods* Red meat and dairy products, especially, are slow to break down and difficult to digest, which only exacerbates an earth element imbalance that results in dampness. Dairy is not a common ingredient in healthy Chinese cuisine and is thought to "injure the spleen."

• *Reduce consumption of coffee, alcohol, and products made from refined flour such as pasta and cookies* All of these foods tend to interfere with proper digestion, which can lead to an increase in dampness and may cause loose stools as well as mental confusion.

• *Don't deprive yourself* Remember that the acts of eating and of preparing food are important aspects of earth energy. Although you must resist the temptation to overeat when it comes to sweets, you should never attempt an excessively strict diet or fasting routine; you'll only end up feeling even more out of balance and out of sorts than ever. A better choice is to prepare a delicious, flavorful, and well-cooked meal, and to eat a small to moderate portion.

• *Look for ways to nourish yourself* To the extent that earth energy responds to nourishment, substitute other nurturing things for food. Perhaps redecorating so that your living space is cozier, buying a sweater that comforts you on a cold night, or pampering yourself with a massage can be the reward that "fills" you.

In addition to emphasizing a healthy diet to treat conditions that derive from an earth energy imbalance, such as irritable bowel syndrome and nausea, an acupuncturist may choose any number of treatments from the Eightfold Path, including acupuncture and herbal remedies.

## Treating Irritable Bowel Syndrome

From a Western perspective, irritable bowel syndrome, or IBS, is a term that describes a variety of conditions that affect the intestines and cause a host of symptoms, including constipation, diarrhea, flatulence, nausea, loss of appetite, and general feelings of lethargy and weakness. There is no known cause of the condition, but doctors believe that stress and the autonomic nervous system, which responds to stress, may play a major role in its development.

A doctor trained in Western medicine would probably run a series of tests, including a rectal exam or sigmoidoscopy, a lower GI (gastrointestinal) series, and various blood tests to check for infection. When these tests come out negative, meaning no other condition or infectious agent is likely to have caused the symptoms, the doctor will diagnose IBS.

As is true for many "modern" medical conditions, IBS lacks a definitive study showing exactly how and why acupuncture helps to treat it. However, some convincing studies support its use. In a 1990 German study by Kunze, Seidel, and Stube, comparing acupuncture with sham treatment, the real acupuncture improved symptoms by 31 percent, compared with 17 percent for the sham treatment. In another study (Diehl, abstracted in the journal *Gastroenterology* in 1994), of ten patients treated with acupuncture, nine improved partially or significantly. In practice, many practitioners combine acupuncture with Chinese herbs, dietary modifications, and other Eightfold Path interventions.

## Treating Gas, Acid, and Ulcers

A number of conditions cause burning in the stomach area and chest; bloating; distension after eating; belching; and difficulty swallowing food. These include nonulcerative dyspepsia (or NUD, also known as heartburn), gastritis, and peptic ulcer disease (PUD). Although their physical symptoms tend to be similar—an acidy feeling in the stomach and throat that spurs sufferers to use (and their doctors to prescribe) common over-the-counter and prescription medications to block acid secretion—there are important distinctions among the conditions. Let's take them one by one:

- Peptic ulcer disease often leads to an ulcer, which is an erosion of the wall of the stomach or the upper intestine. Doctors believe that a bacterial infection of an organism called *Helicobacter pylori* causes most cases of PUD and ulcerative disease.
- Gastritis is an irritation of the stomach membrane; taking aspirin can cause this irritation, as can experiencing high levels of stress, smoking tobacco, and other lifestyle (rather than infectious) factors. These conditions are diagnosed clinically and also by an upper GI series or gastroscopy.
- Nonulcerative dyspepsia, commonly thought of as heartburn and indigestion, is a "functional" illness, which means it is not associated with findings on x-rays or blood tests. A doctor diagnoses NUD based on the patient's symptoms. Some doctors may also put gastrointestinal reflux disorder into this category.

In treating all of these conditions, acupuncture appears to be effective. Many animal and human studies have confirmed that acupuncture moderates the secretion of stomach acid. It does this both by affecting nerve pathways within the brain (which in turn decrease stimulation of acid-producing cells by the vagus nerve) and by affecting the hormones involved in stomach-acid secretion. For instance, several studies have suggested that acupuncture can aid in the treatment of peptic ulcer disease. In one study by Kajdos (*American Journal of Acupuncture*, 1977), of seventy-one patients with ulcers who were treated with acupuncture, 63 percent had very good responses, and 28 percent experienced temporary relief. Other studies have used experimental and animal models to demonstrate positive effects of acupuncture on ulcers (Lux et al., *Gut*, 1994; Jin et al., *American Journal of Physiology*, 1996). However, no laboratory has yet performed the definitive study that irrefutably demonstrates this effect.

Several clinical reports in the literature demonstrate the efficacy of acupuncture in treating NUD as well. (A fuller discussion can be found in Diehl, *Journal of Alternative and Complementary Medicine* 5 [1], 1999.) Since NUD and other functional problems are related to many factors, including diet, stress, and a sensitivity of the nervous system to bloating of the stomach, Chinese medicine, which addresses illness and health in a holistic way, is a particularly good system to treat such conditions.

In addition, some acupuncture studies show great benefit to patients suffering from achalasia, or difficulty in swallowing. Scientists believe that the condition involves a muscular ring at the lower esophagus that, because of a neurological and hormonal imbalance, becomes abnormally tight. Acupuncture can help relax the esophageal sphincter, which diminishes the symptoms of achalasia (Guelrud, *Digestive Diseases and Sciences*, 1991).

Another possible use of acupuncture for digestive problems is to stimulate gastrointestinal activity after surgery. Anyone who has had abdominal surgery knows that moving gas and stool through the intestines is a good sign that the body is mending after the procedure. When this does not happen, the condition is called postoperative ileus. Several studies have indicated that acupuncture is useful in preventing this dangerous outcome.

## *Treating Nausea and Vomiting*

As chronicled in earlier chapters, the National Institutes of Health Scientific Consensus Conference Report of 1997 cited studies confirming that nausea and vomiting during pregnancy (one such study was published by Dundee and McMillan, in *Acupuncture Electrotherapeutics*, 1990), postoperatively (Al-Sadi et al., *Anaesthesia*, 1997), and in association with chemotherapy (a more recent study by Shen et al. was published in the *Journal of the American Medical Association*, 2000) are symptoms for which acupuncture is effective. Unlike most of the other studies on acupuncture, many of the nausea and vomiting studies have been well controlled, randomized, and carefully designed, so that the mainstream medical community trusts their results.

Frequently, the studies used stomach 36, a point that when stimulated with acupuncture quiets the "rebellious *qi*" of the stomach (which is how Chinese medicine views nausea and vomiting). Another commonly used point was pericardium 6, on the inside of the wrist. This point is sometimes called the "seasick point," since massaging it will calm the nausea associated with seasickness. In fact, you can purchase bands called seasick bands at drugstores. These soft bracelets massage pericardium 6, and anyone suffering with nausea—from pregnant women to chemotherapy patients to seagoing voyagers—can gain relief by wearing one.

✸

## *Restoring Earth Energy Flow with Acupuncture*

In addition to the points mentioned in connection to the specific conditions just discussed, the following acupuncture points are among those commonly used to treat earth energy imbalances:

• *Conception Vessel 12 ("middle duct")* Treating this point, halfway between the bottom of the breastbone and the belly button, helps restore balance in the digestive organs, including the stomach and spleen. Initially, food will move more quickly and efficiently through the digestive system, helping to relieve cramping, bloating, and gas. The heaviness and lethargy that people with earth energy imbalances feel will dissipate as treatment continues.

• *Spleen 6 ("three* yin *junction")* This point gets its familiar name from the *yin* channels of the leg that join here on the inside of the calf. If your acupuncturist focuses on this point, you may find that you have fewer cravings for sweets, more energy, and greater ability to digest efficiently.

• *Stomach 40 ("abundant splendor")* Sometimes called the "cornucopia point," this point on the belly of the large shin muscle helps you to cut through dampness and get the full bounty from life. It harmonizes the stomach and spleen and can physically help sluggishness, heavy legs, and bloating.

## Maintaining Your Great Brightness

Your nurturing earth energy is precious. However, if you match the key descriptions in this chapter, you probably spend so much time taking care of others—feeding them, providing sound advice, offering a kind of balance and equilibrium to the swirling world around you—that you forget to tend to your own needs and thus risk energy imbalance. Especially during the changes of seasons, when energy is in a transitional phase, you must take time to relax, to feed your own soul and body, to clear your thoughts, and to maintain a clear, fluid (rather than stuck and impassable) energy. By doing so, not only will you help keep your particularly vulnerable digestive system in good working order, but also your entire being will feel freer and better able to remain in balance.

In addition to the important dietary tips previously mentioned, here are a few suggestions that should help you nurture your earth energy:

• *Exercise* Movement is the best way to clear dampness, and many acupuncture points, such as one along the spleen channel called the "earth motivator," help to create movement in the earth channels when stimulated. You can get your energy moving in the right direction by exercising regularly. If you have an earth imbalance, your acupuncturist will undoubtedly recommend taking a twenty- to thirty-minute walk each morning, bicycling, dancing, or any other active physical exercise. Yoga exercises are also encouraged.

• *Herbal remedies* Your acupuncturist may well devise an individualized herbal routine for you, depending on your specific needs, body type, and symptoms, in addition to your earth energy basics. One of the most helpful herbs for earth types is ginger, which is also good for relieving nausea and vomiting. Licorice is also a popular Chinese herb for digestion and is frequently added to formulas to make the other herbs easier on the stomach.

A common herbal combination that gets rid of dampness and harmonizes the spleen and stomach is called *sausorea amomum six gentlemen.* The first two herbs dry the dampness, while the herbs known collectively as "six gentlemen"—ginseng, atractylodes, poria, licorice, citrus peel, and pinellia—form a common earth-treatment herbal regimen. This combination helps balance metabolism, increase energy, and improve digestion.

• Qi gong *exercise for earth* Qi gong provides another easy way of strengthening the earth energy. The simplest spleen *qi gong* is performed by placing the hands, one over the other, on the belly (around conception vessel 12; see the previous section) and massaging the area in a clockwise direction around the belly button, feeling the warmth permeate the center.

By working with your acupuncturist, and learning to listen to and heed your body's signals and needs, you can maintain your center and your health as a powerful member of the earth energy family.

8

# METAL
## The Very Great Abyss

THE CRISP, PRISTINE FEEL OF a fall day in New England captures the experience of the metal element. In the autumn, nature is paring down to what is essential. The leaves are turning and dropping, and the bare structure of the tree branches begins to show from beneath. Growth in the garden has stopped, and whatever has not been harvested is rotting and becoming food for next year's growth. Even the sounds of autumn are different from what has come before. Whereas summer air buzzes with activity, fall is a quieter time, in which one can walk along a path of fallen leaves and listen to their crispness underfoot.

In the creative cycle of Chinese medicine, the metal element symbolizes this feeling of quietness and a return to something simpler—the feeling of "letting go." Just as nature lets go of the busyness and bloom of summer as the autumn arrives, so too should we humans let go of our busyness, of our youth, and of the nonessential trappings of our world as we emerge into the later part of our lives. Metal is associated with the later years of our lives, when it's common to turn inward, to become introspective, and to seek less outwardly for our enjoyment. Someone who has always sought exciting but temporary relationships might "settle down" with a life partner. Someone else who has tried to accumulate showy, expensive jewelry or artwork might turn instead to philanthropy. It's equally common for previously secular individuals to begin to seek a more spiritual or religious connection in their later years.

In some people, the later years might imply a quiet wisdom and confidence that comes with age and experience. In others, there might be regret or even sadness over missed opportunities and lost loved ones. In the autumn of our years, there is a sense of clarity and quality that is universal.

This same sense of quality expresses itself in someone with metal energy, no matter what his or her age. Metal seeks quality, purity, and perfection that may take the form of choosing the right clothes at all times or decorating one's house with care. Someone with a strongly expressed metal energy may take special care to choose exactly the right words with which to express his or her ideas. Since the quality of metal is of turning inward, there is a depth to metal people, a place within them that can't be accessed by other people. The image of someone quietly at prayer in a medieval cathedral evokes the solitary strength of metal energy.

Metal is also associated with the heavens, or the Father archetype. Sometimes, a person with a strong metal energy is involved in an actual fatherly relationship, particularly with or as a father who represents some of the aspects of the metal element. Other people with metal energy might seek to bring a strong leader, a guru or a teacher, into their lives, someone who displays typical paternal attributes such as authority, structure, or protection.

## Metal Energy in Health and Disease

The organs related to the metal element are the lungs (the *yin* organ) and the large intestine, or colon (the *yang* organ). The lungs inhale pure air, which mixes with nutritive *qi* from the stomach to provide the *qi* that runs through our meridians and nourishes every cell of the body. The large intestine is the organ that lets go of the waste. Between these two organs, there is a constant balance between the taking in of breath, freshness, and inspiration and the letting go of what clutters our lives and bodies with matter we no longer need.

Just as the large intestine, or colon, has to let go and relax in order to release physical waste products, people have to dispel and expel what they no longer need emotionally and intellectually. In all aspects of our existence, we need to let go and loosen up, in order to have a life that functions relatively smoothly and in a relaxed way. The expression "anal retentive" is a common description of people who are too uptight and rigid in their approach to their daily lives, a personality trait particularly associated with metal. Someone obsessed with cleanliness, neatness, and precision has a strong—perhaps imbalanced—metal energy.

Think of the character of Dr. Niles Crane in the television show "Frasier." Concerned with status and refinement, he is constantly rigid and tense about obtaining and achieving the "very best." As we watch him, we're tempted to psychoanalyze this television psychiatrist ourselves. Apparently, he feels that he's inferior to his brother and, because of his effete manner, that he's a disappointment to his father. These feelings often lead him to focus on external objects of quality—his art collection, his furniture, his fine wines—to define him, which is one way that an imbalance of metal energy may manifest itself.

The other end of the metal spectrum represents remarkable strength and confidence. When Nelson Mandela was released from his decades of imprisonment in South Africa, he emerged with an unforgettable proud bearing. His posture was erect and strong, and his demeanor was that of nobility. His face was relaxed, though it projected a sadness. No one who watched could have been unmoved by his solemn presence and by the witnessing of a strong, powerful—and balanced—metal energy.

Throughout most cultures, heaven represents this concept of purity and perfection. The lungs, which receive energy (air) from the heavens, are the primary organs of the metal energy. They are paired with the large intestine to complete the cycle of taking in purity and eliminating impurity.

## *The Receiver of Pure* Qi

The lungs are considered the receiver of pure *qi* from the heavens. That is, the lungs inhale pure air, which is mixed with nutritive *qi* from the stomach to provide the *qi* that runs through our meridians. In a way, you can imagine the lungs as the organs that govern the relationship between the internal and external; along with the large intestine, the lungs organize and distribute the good things we take in from the outside. The pathway of the lung (upper *tai yin*) meridian begins under the clavicle bone and then branches deep into the lung. The surface meridian crosses the front of the shoulder and continues down the surface of the arm to the thumb (see Figure 2).

The lungs protect the body from outside harm by controlling the *wei qi*, the protective energy that surrounds us, and also by their connection to the skin. In addition to taking in essential oxygen, the steady, rhythmic nature of breathing helps to control the autonomic nervous system, calming the body after a period of excitement or preparing it for action when danger or other stress arises. This relationship between breathing and the nervous system forms the basis for meditation, yoga, and *qi gong* breathing exercises.

Even within the Western paradigm, the lungs perform this function. Certain parts of the respiratory system—the tiny hairs in the nose and the bronchi (breathing tubes) in the lungs themselves—prevent harmful substances from entering the body. Then, by taking in oxygen and distributing it throughout the body, the lungs bring to each cell the energy it needs to survive and thrive.

The skin, which "breathes" through its pores, is also considered part of the lungs in Chinese medicine. In addition, the skin plays a protective role for the body by forming the first line of defense against external environmental hazards and also by helping to maintain proper body temperature through perspiration and shivering—again, through its pores. When the metal energy becomes imbalanced, conditions related to the lungs and the skin, such as asthma and eczema, often emerge.

### The Minister of Elimination of Waste

The *yang* organ of the metal element is the large intestine, responsible for the collection and excretion of waste products. The large intestine (upper *yang ming*) channel begins at the index finger and traverses the forearm, running across the shoulder and up the side of the neck, where it ends beside the nostril (see Figure 6 on page 140 and Figure 3 in Chapter 6). Acupuncturists often use this channel to treat tennis elbow, a form of tendinitis that causes recurrent pain on the outside of the upper forearm below the crease of the elbow. The large intestine plays a major role in the balance and purity of bodily substances. Its health depends on the proper functioning of the lungs, in that the breath helps to regulate digestion by regulating abdominal pressure. That's why you'll find that taking deep and regular breaths, as well as practicing deep-breathing exercise regularly, will help prevent and treat constipation.

When the metal energy becomes imbalanced, the person often develops a feeling of impurity or inadequacy, or even of being damaged. These feelings arise when the large intestine does not perform its elimination function, which may also lead to the equally common metal need for external structures or for other people to define oneself.

## Metal Energy Out of Balance

I had a patient, a CEO of a company, who came in with a shoulder problem (not coincidentally, manifesting as pain experienced over the metal

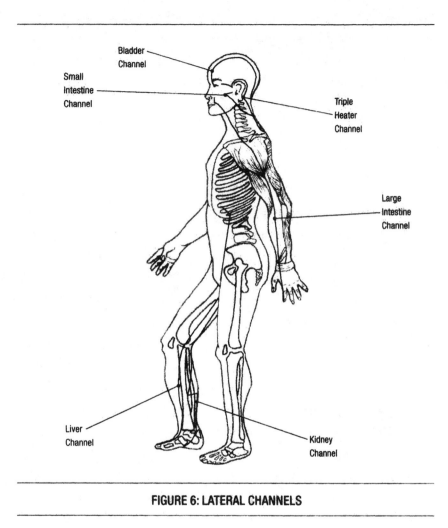

**FIGURE 6: LATERAL CHANNELS**

meridians of the arm). At each visit, he would wait until I was in the room and then slowly remove his Rolex watch, his large gold ring, his bulging money clip, and his state-of-the-art cell phone, and then tell me how much his company was worth that day. Only with repeated questioning and discussion did I find out how empty this man's life really was. It was as if he were saying, "Here's what my value is; don't look further." Often, this is the emotional pattern that arises when metal energy is out of balance.

Another way someone with a metal energy might reveal an imbalance is by adopting an external construct—a religious belief, a political idea, or a lifestyle—to define himself or herself. For instance, some people are "religious" about macrobiotics, so much so that they view the world through this lens. Other people use an illness to define themselves. One of my patients has chronic fatigue (also called CFIDS, chronic fatigue and immune dysfunction syndrome). She is seemingly unable to separate herself from her illness. When asked about her personal relationships, she answers, "CFIDS people have a lot of trouble with relationships." She even sees a sprained ankle as a manifestation of her illness. It is as if she has no internal sense of value or self, just the external trappings of her illness.

Someone with metal energy out of balance may even seem to be perpetually grieving. Here, the voice has the sound quality associated with metal, called weeping in Chinese medicine. It is a sad voice, frequently quiet and cracking, but this tenor exists even when the person is speaking of neutral or positive experiences. While it is natural to evidence a sad voice when speaking of sad things or when truly grieving, someone with a metal energy imbalance projects grief and sadness inappropriately, as a manifestation of the imbalance itself. For instance, I recently had a sad middle-aged patient who dated the beginning of her colitis to around the time of her father's death. When I asked when he died, she answered in a grief-stricken whisper, "1972."

The physical conditions that emerge when there is an imbalance of metal energy include eczema and other skin problems, especially early in life, as well as chronic respiratory problems such as sinusitis and asthma. Since the energy in the meridian tends to cycle from the liver to the lungs at about 3:00 A.M. every night, someone with excess liver energy and/or deficient lung energy may wake up at that time and experience respiratory problems, such as wheezing or sneezing. In later life, such people often develop colitis or irritable bowel syndrome, a problem of the large intestine. Diarrhea can occur frequently at 5:00 to 7:00 A.M., when energy has moved from the lungs into the large intestine.

Furthermore, as discussed in Chapter 2, an imbalance of one element will often disrupt others. Because metal feeds the water element in the creative cycle, if metal energy becomes imbalanced, problems of water deficiency may arise, such as fatigue, kidney disorders, and back pain. When metal fails to control wood energy via the control cycle, problems related to excess wood such as headaches, musculoskeletal injuries, and pelvic disorders may develop.

# Treating Metal Energy Imbalance

If you have metal energy problems, you and your practitioner will work together to bring your energy back into balance. The climate condition most associated with metal is dryness, which can appear as the dryness in the lungs that accompanies bronchitis and asthma, as dry skin, or as constipation, which is dryness in the colon. Thus, proper hydration is important for proper metal function. So too is breathing, as the breath brings the life force into the body.

### *Breathing Life:* Qi Gong

No matter what energy type you are within the Five-Element paradigm, correct breathing—meaning deep, controlled, and regular—is essential to good health and balance. This is especially true if you are a metal energy type, since so much depends on the clear and proper functioning of the lung and the large intestine meridians. Chinese medicine has developed a series of breathing exercises within *qi gong* practice. These exercises help to strengthen the lungs as well as increase energy and help to still the metal mind, which tends to be perfectionist and obsessive when its energy is out of balance.

Before you can start to practice these exercises, you must learn to breathe correctly. Yes, that's right—you may have to relearn an automatic function you've been performing on your own for all of your life! The truth is that most Westerners fail to use all of their breathing muscles to their fullest, which leaves the diaphragm and the abdomen—the two prime breathing pumps—underused and the body underexposed to the full amount of oxygen it requires. That's why *qi gong* practice often concentrates on deep abdominal breathing techniques. Other exercises include reverse abdominal breathing, lung breathing, body breathing, and palm and sole breathing.

To get started, try these two simple exercises:

• *Abdominal breathing* Also known as diaphragmatic breathing, this method is the one primarily used in *qi gong* and meditation. Although diaphragmatic breathing may take some time to master, the benefits are well worth the effort. Start by lying down on the floor. Put one hand on your chest and the other on your abdomen. As you inhale deeply through your nose, try filling your abdomen with air (which will expand and move the hand upon it) while keeping your chest flat (and that hand immobile). As you exhale through your mouth, watch as your abdomen deflates. By breathing this way, you're using the diaphragm and abdomen as breathing pumps. You're drawing the breath deep down into the bottom of the lungs—the *yin* phase of breathing, which draws energy into the body and through the meridians—and on exhalation, which is the *yang* phase, pushing the energy toward the skin and muscles.

• Qi gong *breathing for metal energy* Here is a *qi gong* exercise specifically designed to strengthen the lungs and help the process of elimination. Relax and stand with your feet shoulder-width apart. Hold your hands, palms facing each other, at eye level. Take a breath. Then, thrust your hands down so that they wind up at your sides. While thrusting the hands, exhale rapidly, saying the word "shah." You'll find that this empties your lungs and facilitates all aspects of the "letting-go" process.

If you visit an acupuncturist and have symptoms related to metal energy out of balance, such as respiratory problems or persistent skin conditions, the practitioner will likely emphasize building proper breathing exercises like the ones described here as well as other treatments derived from the Eightfold Path Toward Health. The following sections review the efficacy of acupuncture for treating some specific illnesses related to metal energy.

## Treating Asthma and Other Respiratory Problems

More than 10 million Americans suffer from asthma, a condition characterized by wheezing, difficulty in breathing, tightness in the chest, and coughing up of excess mucus. These symptoms arise, Western scientists believe, when the bronchial tubes in the lungs become inflamed and hyperactive, often due to an allergic reaction to any number of substances, such as pet dander, pollen, or mold spores. Other triggers of asthma attacks include respiratory infections and exercise. Treatment of asthma typically includes steroids that help reduce inflammation and drugs called bronchodilators that act to open up tight and clogged bronchial tubes, thus making it easier for the asthma sufferer to breathe.

Within the traditional Chinese medicine paradigm, the causes and treatment of wheezing and other breathing problems that look like asthma in the West are much more complicated and intricate. In fact, there isn't even a word for *asthma* in Chinese. The symptoms can have external causes such as wind and cold attacking the lungs, or internal causes such as weakness of the kidneys or inability of the spleen to transform phlegm, leading to congestion. Any imbalance within the meridian system can disrupt the metal energy, causing respiratory problems similar to the symptoms of asthma.

Several studies indicate that acupuncture can help improve feelings of general well-being as well as reduce the need for conventional medication in patients with asthma, acute rhinitis (runny and itchy nose, related to allergies), and chronic sinusitis, especially when applied in combination with conventional medication. A 1991 study in *Thorax* and a 1996 study in the *Journal of Alternative and Complementary Medicine* both involved patients whose asthma symptoms improved after they underwent acupuncture treatments. In a 1982 study of eighteen chronic sinusitis patients published in the *American Journal of Chinese Medicine*, patients who received acupuncture treatments fared far better than did those who received either antibiotics or laser therapy after just six sessions.

How does acupuncture alleviate symptoms of asthma and other respiratory problems? There are three main theories. First, acupuncture appears to work in a way similar to bronchodilators, by relaxing the bronchial tubes and thus making it easier for patients to breathe. Acupuncture also works to reduce inflammation by triggering the production of a body chemical called adrenocorticotropic hormone (ACTH), which in turn produces cortisol, a type of steroid—a natural counterpart to the conventional prescription drugs so often prescribed by physicians to their asthma patients. Finally, according to a meta-analysis of several studies published in a 2000 issue of the *Journal of Alternative and Complementary Medicine*, acupuncture treatments were shown to stimulate the production of certain immune-system cells. These cells moderate the body's allergic response, thus lessening the wheezing and runny nose associated with asthma and allergic rhinitis.

## Treating Dermatitis, Eczema, and Other Skin Problems

A condition called "neurodermatitis" in many Chinese texts is actually two conditions here in the West: eczema and dermatitis. Eczema is a skin condition that results in patches of dry, extremely itchy, thickened skin. It often occurs first in childhood and usually affects the skin behind the knees and in the folds of the elbow. About a third of those who suffer with eczema have respiratory allergies such as asthma and hay fever. Dermatitis consists of an itchy rash of small bumps, blisters, and general swelling. Some people with dermatitis also suffer a burning sensation in the eyes and nose. Dermatitis is caused by hypersensitivity—an allergy—to any number of substances that is triggered by direct contact with plants, chemicals, metals, or drugs.

Treatment of both conditions here in the West usually includes use of corticosteroid creams to reduce inflammation and swelling. If the condition is related to allergies, as is often the case with eczema and dermatitis, doctors often prescribe antihistamines, drugs that act to moderate the allergic response.

As is true so often when it comes to Western studies of Chinese medical techniques, studies concerning the efficacy of acupuncture for skin conditions are relatively few and far between. The only controlled study to date took place under laboratory conditions in which scientists triggered the development of itchy skin in their subjects and then tested various treatments. What they found bolstered the results of smaller, uncontrolled studies and anecdotal evidence: acupuncture appears to reduce itching and inflammation by inhibiting the release of histamine, the chemical the body produces during allergic reactions. The results of this 1984 study, published in *Dermatologica Venereologica*, indicate that acupuncture treatment alleviates symptoms sooner and keeps them at bay longer than no treatment or treatment with sham acupuncture.

Furthermore, several well-controlled studies show that certain Chinese herb treatments alleviate symptoms of dermatitis and eczema. Specifically, in a 1992 study and 1994 follow-up printed in the *British Journal of Dermatology*, thirty-seven children with allergic eczema were treated with Chinese herbs in a double-blind placebo-controlled trial, meaning that neither the patients nor the doctors knew whether any given child was getting the herbs or the placebo. Eighteen children exhibited more than 90 percent recovery, and five more had partial responses. A similar randomized controlled study on adults, published in 1995 in *Clinical and Experimental Dermatology*, showed similarly significant improvement with Chinese herbal treatment.

## Restoring Metal Energy Flow with Acupuncture

If an acupuncturist concludes that your metal energy needs to be addressed, he or she will probably treat you and your symptoms with a full complement of methods from the Eightfold Path, including acupuncture, breathing exercises, and herbal medicine. In addition to choosing specific acupoints to alleviate particular symptoms, your acupuncturist may needle the following points to treat your metal energy:

• *Lung 7 ("meridian gutter")* As its familiar name implies, this point is used to purify and cleanse the metal meridians. Located on the inside of the wrist over the bony process just below the thumb, it is a junction (*luo*) point between the lung and large intestine. Practitioners often use it to activate some Extraordinary Meridians. As explained in Chapter 2, these eight channels are actually made up of points from other meridians and act as storehouses of *yin* and *yang* energy.

• *Large intestine 4 ("joining of the valleys")* Known in Chinese as *ho kou*, this acupoint is perhaps the best known on the body. Found in the notch between the thumb and forefinger, it is often used by acupuncturists to treat pain. In Five-Element acupuncture, it is the source point of the large intestine. Needling this point helps trigger "letting go," either of physical things such as waste products blocked by constipation, or emotions such as grief. Bringing on a menstrual period or simply encouraging an internal cleansing may also be affected through this point.

• *Lung 9 ("very great abyss")* The evocative moniker of this point suggests its function, which is to take someone through the depths of grief to a place of healing. Physically, it is used to marshal the essence of the metal energy, since it is the source point of the lung channel, located over the radial artery at the wrist crease.

• *Large intestine 20 ("welcome fragrance")* This point beside the nostril is the last point on the metal channels before energy enters the stomach. Thus, as its familiar name implies, it represents the successful elim- ination of waste and the ability that elimination engenders to receive the fragrance and bounty that is associated with the earth energy, which directly precedes metal in the creative cycle.

# Maintaining a Healthy Balance and Internal Rhythm

Metal energy is one that thrives on balance—between what's outside and what it lets in, between self-reflection and the tendency to grieve or become depressed, between order and chaos. Here are a few a tips to keep your metal energy strong and healthy:

• *Maintain clarity and simplicity—within reason* A strong need for clarity is part of your nature, so why fight it? Don't clutter your life with needless appointments, papers, and obligations. Create a clear and work- able bookkeeping system, find proper places for all of your belongings, and set up a balanced schedule that works for you and your family. At the same time, don't let your need for order overwhelm you or the peo- ple you love. Life will never be perfect, and the universe is naturally dis- ordered, so do your breathing exercises every day, and let these disruptions go.

• *Eat well and on a regular schedule* If your metal energy is imbal- anced, you may tend to skip meals, because you simply don't much care for food; it just doesn't interest you as much as it does, say, a more earth- expressed person. On the other hand, you may be a gourmet, focusing on the highest quality of food presentation, fine wines, and exotic cui- sine. Unfortunately, both extremes can lead to nutritional depletion. Talk to your acupuncturist about developing a healthy diet for you, one that will help entice your appetite and your sense of quality while pro- viding your body with the nutrients it needs to survive and thrive.

• *Humidify your environment* Keeping the air rich with moisture helps maintain a strong, balanced lung energy. Even in Western medicine, doctors advise patients to use a humidifier in dry situations, particularly during the winter when closed heating systems use up moisture. Drying the lungs and breathing passages can suppress the immune protection of those tissues.

• *Enjoy herbal remedies* Moistening the lungs and eliminating cough and mucus are common goals of lung herbs in Chinese medicine. One formula, called upright *qi* powder, is made of three herbs—Korean ginseng, schizandra, and ophiopogon—and is most commonly added to other herbal remedies by skilled herbalists. Elecampane and red clover are also common herbs given to treat lung problems. Other expectorant herbs include pinellia and apricot seed (in small doses). The most common lung herb is mahuang, or ephedra, and should be used only under supervision, as it can cause cardiac problems when used incorrectly. Your acupuncturist will prescribe the right herbal combination for you.

# 9

# WATER
## Greater Mountain Stream

I ONCE HAD SQUIRRELS IN my attic. They were chewing through my eaves and storing their winter's nuts above my bedroom, and not at all quietly. The exterminator plugged the holes and then lead-lined the gutters and eaves. It was late September, and the squirrels were cut off from their food stores. Panic set in, and for the next few weeks, squirrels ran about in terror throughout my yard. They knew that the cold weather was coming and that their careful plans had been disrupted.

According to Chinese medical philosophy, the body contains a special place to store reserves of energy. It is a place that can either provide the strength to push through obstacles or become the seat of fear and of depletion. That place is called the kidney. The kidneys are one organ of the water element; the other is the bladder. The bladder is a reservoir where the waters of the body collect and then, once catalyzed by the *qi*, are eliminated.

Water energy also involves the concept of power. The power of water is evident in nature. It carved the Grand Canyon, turns deserts into lush vineyards, and capsizes mighty ships with a shrug. The gentle waves of the ocean, a hard rainfall, and a river rushing by its banks also express the idea of power and energy.

In life, our power comes from a feeling of being rooted, connected to something solid. Even martial arts masters bend their knees a bit to lower their center of gravity in order to connect themselves to the earth and become more "immovable" and thus stronger and better able to meet challenges. Power also comes from courage, from valor. Someone who is courageous is able to perform tasks that are otherwise out of the question. And power also comes from an awareness of one's strengths and one's limitations.

Finally, power comes from wisdom. The kidneys are the storehouse of wisdom, which consists not merely of intelligent thoughts but also of the kind of age-old knowledge that guides our proper behavior. Wisdom, of course, is traditionally associated with being elderly, and as we age, we develop wisdom (it is hoped) that both informs our own actions and teaches those around us. Humans live longer than most other species, perhaps because we're exposed to elders who, after having experienced danger and lived through it, help us to avoid those dangers and live to an old age ourselves. This relationship of aging to wisdom is an expression of water energy.

Part of the power of the water element is sexual potency. Sexual intimacy relates more to the fire element (see Chapter 6), but the act itself, for both men and women, relates to the kidneys. Low kidney energy may trigger both an inability to become sexually aroused and low sexual performance. Infertility and low sperm counts are manifestations of low kidney energy.

Psychologically speaking, water energy relates to both fear and courage. Someone with strong water energy can have a lot of drive and a seemingly endless well of energy from which to draw. These types may need less sleep and be able to party longer than those around them, staying oddly young and vital even as the years roll by. Cyclist Lance Armstrong, for example, won his personal battle with cancer and now perpetually leads the way—not only in the long-distance bicycle race, the Tour de France, but also for all of us in our day-to-day lives. Armstrong has strong water energy.

Water people may have a lot of sexual energy. In fact, the herbal shops in Chinatowns across the world are frequented by men looking for supposed secrets of potency, and what they are given are herbal tonics for the kidney energy. Whether the tonics work as potency potions is questionable, but their goal is to increase the kidney *yang*, the energy that drives potency and performance.

On the other hand, the water element also involves stillness and depth, much as water seeks the deepest level in nature. Strong water energy can therefore be present in someone who has a quiet internal strength that may not even show at first. Someone with strong water energy is not necessarily the most vocal nor most visible but is the one who'll come through during the tough times. He or she is the person on whom others will come to rely.

## Water Energy in Health and Disease

Winter is water's season, the time of the year when the entire natural world—including the squirrels in my attic that scurried desperately to find and store food—contracts and condenses, living on its stores of energy until the season of growth and renewal begins. Without reserves of energy, both squirrels and humans become more vulnerable to disease and depletion.

When one of my patients came for her first appointment, she had a disabling illness that limited her ability to move. Despite her physical restrictions, she was studying for two master's degrees in two different states, refusing to allow her disability to stunt her life or her potential in any way. This woman's courage and drive, and her refusal to give in or even to acknowledge her illness, are good examples of strong water energy, complete with a fearlessness that may not be completely appropriate. Frequently in Chinese medicine, a person's strengths and challenges mirror one another, with the same strong quality leading both to benefits (such as a healthy sense of determination) and disadvantages (such as recklessness).

## The Minister of Power and Bodily Fluids

In Chinese medicine, the kidneys are considered the body's most important reservoir of essential energy. Although the concept of reserves is not one that Western medicine typically embraces, you can think of it in terms of emotional and physical strength and endurance. A weight lifter who squeezes out one more repetition, an athlete who has an extra kick at the end of a race, a businessperson who stays up most of the night to finish a proposal, and a pregnant woman giving one more push after an exhausting and lengthy labor all exhibit physical and psychological reserves.

According to Chinese medicine, we come into this world with a certain amount of life force, called *jing*, that buffers us from the wear and tear of life. People born with bountiful *jing* are those who seem able to go and go for ninety years, never ill or incapacitated, seemingly with endless amounts of energy. Those who seem to be sickly from birth or before, and who tend to be susceptible to lots of physical or emotional illness and stress, are those with deficient *jing*.

From a Western perspective, the water-energy *yin* organ, the kidneys, acts to regulate the amount of water and other substances in the blood and to remove wastes from the blood through the urine. Several thousand quarts of blood pass through the kidneys every day for filtration. However, the organ closest to the Chinese medicine concept of the kidneys in Western medicine is not the kidney but the small endocrine organ that sits on top of it.

Called adrenal because it is on top of the kidney (renal) organ, this gland secretes a number of hormones important to the way the body responds to stress. Aldosterone, for instance, is a hormone that helps maintain blood pressure by retaining salt in the body, while adrenaline (also known as epinephrine) responds acutely to stress, pumping blood through our veins at a rapid rate and readying us for fight or flight. Cortisol, a slower responder to stress, increases blood sugar, reduces inflammation, and cushions other physiological responses to any kind of physical or emotional stress. Dihydroepiandosterone is a storage hormone, able to convert itself into other hormones as the body requires. Together, these adrenal hormones work to direct the body's response to stress.

The kidney channel, or lower *shao yin*, starts on the sole of the foot at a point called "bubbling spring," where the *qi* "bubbles" up from the earth into the body (see Figure 2 in Chapter 6 and Figure 6 in Chapter 8). It ascends the inside of the leg and thigh, through the groin, and up the anterior chest near the midline, ending below the clavicle. The upper kidney points, on the chest, have particular significance. They have names such as "spirit storehouse" and "burial ground of the spirit" and are used when any energy imbalance involves the spirit (see Chapter 6).

## The Minister of the Reservoir

Where the kidneys are the source of the power of water, the bladder is the organ that stores it. Without storage, energy will easily run out, and fatigue and lack of energy result. People who tire easily frequently also have to urinate a lot, as if their bladders were smaller.

The bladder (lower *tai yang*) channel is the largest channel in the body. (See Figure 4 in Chapter 6.) It begins at the internal corner of the eye, a point known as bladder 1, or "eye bright." It traverses the head and continues down the back of the neck (through bladder 10, known as "heavenly pillar"). It descends the back near the spine, until reaching the sacrum, along what is termed the inner bladder line. It then goes internal and comes out at the top of the back again, descending along the inside of the scapula and downward along the outer bladder line. It then crosses the buttocks, descends the back of the thigh and the outside of the legs, and ends at the small toe.

Several inner bladder line points on the back have particular significance. Called *shu* points (or associated effect points), they exist on the bladder channel but actually connect directly to the twelve organs. There is one *shu* point for each organ and function, as well as *shu* points for other structures such as the diaphragm, bones, and blood. The outer bladder line also has points that correspond to each of the twelve organs, but they pertain to the more psycho-spiritual aspects of these organs. For instance, "spirit hall" (bladder 39) relates to the heart and to bladder 15, the heart *shu* point; "earth granary" (bladder 45) relates to the stomach and is opposite bladder 21, the stomach *shu* point.

## Water Energy Out of Balance

The water element is where we see many of the chronic conditions that our bodies display in reaction to stress. When prolonged conditions exhaust us, the kidney and bladder pulses weaken, which causes the fluids of the body to dry up. When that occurs, there is "heat," which can manifest itself as inflammation in almost any part of the body, causing red and itchy eyes, a sore and scratchy throat, or inflammation of joints and muscles, among other conditions. It can manifest itself as exhaustion, the inability to perform one more task or to deal with one more situation.

Impotence, lack of libido, and difficulty in performing the sex act itself may also stem from a disruption in water energy. In fact, one aspect of Chinese medicine that is almost nonexistent in the West is the premise that too much sexual activity will exhaust the reserves. Although one theory holds that this doctrine is a means to encourage birth control, more common interpretations identify the kidneys as the source of the "spark" of sexual energy, and thus excess sexual activity will deplete the reserves that these organs have stored. *Jing* itself frequently refers to sexual energy, particularly in regard to young people, whose reserves are plentiful, and thus young people without strong sexual desire are sometimes said to have low *jing*.

In older people, the *jing* has much to do with the wisdom that comes with age; thus, a weakness of the water element can reveal itself in someone's inability or unwillingness to age gracefully. A sixty-year-old woman in a tight miniskirt and a man with dyed hair and a penchant for chasing young women can be examples of kidney energy imbalance. In addition, a water element imbalance can manifest itself through feelings of extreme vulnerability and the fear that there's nothing left to protect us. Such feelings can lead to depression, lack of motivation, and even loss of a will to live. The need for periods of quiet self-reflection, so healthy when it helps focus the energy on intellectual and philosophical pursuits, may turn into irritable isolation, cynicism, and inflexibility.

A long-running commercial for an insurance company promoted a "piece of the rock," linking the company with an image of eternal solidity. Imagine having this quiet solidity internally and the feelings of rootedness and strength it would bring. Now imagine what it would be like to have no internal solidity, to be buffeted about like a twig in a roaring river; this is akin to the fear that a weak water element may engender. We see fear in other elements (the personal vulnerability of a fire imbalance or the frustrated anxiety of wood), but the fear associated with a water imbalance is a fear at the core, in the bones.

Someone with water imbalance, then, may suffer from panic attacks and severe fatigue, as well as backaches and pain in the knees where the bladder channel passes. The symptoms may include frequent urination and thirst, as well as a seeming loss of will to push through difficult situations. An example is a patient who came to my office with the diagnosis of panic disorder but insisted that he had no psychological reason to be so anxious. After a lengthy examination, he revealed that he had been working day and night on a project for months before this, had missed sleep, and drank lots of coffee (which is dehydrating) without other fluids. Only after this period of overwork and overstress did he begin having panic attacks. He had, in fact, exhausted his kidney reserves and thus was filled with fear as his water imbalance grew. Treating his water element with acupuncture and herbs helped to eliminate his panic attacks.

Many of my patients have chronic fatigue, either from chronic illnesses or from chronic fatigue syndrome. Although other problems may coexist, these patients also suffer from a deficiency of water energy. In physical terms, this means that they have no ability to cope with physical exertion without becoming exhausted, and they have no reserve of energy. Emotionally, these patients tend to be exhausted as well, unable to cope with changes in their lives. Panic disorder is common. The fight-or-flight response is overactive, causing them to startle easily and to be sensitive to noise. There can be thirst or a craving for salt (the taste associated with the water element). Also, as the bladder energy is depleted, there is an inability to hold any reserves, with frequent urination and backaches common.

## Treating Water Energy Imbalance

If your water is imbalanced and you suffer from one or more of the conditions outlined in the preceding section, you and your Chinese medicine practitioner will collaborate to bring your water energy back into balance. If your water energy is excessive, your body and your soul may become hardened and inflexible, leading to conditions such as arthritis and urinary problems. If your resources have become depleted, you'll feel worn down and overwhelmed, and you may suffer from such conditions as chronic fatigue, loss of libido, and depression.

Many symptoms can result from water imbalances. Depleted water can fail to control the fire element, leading to palpitations and hot flashes. This is commonly what happens in menopause. Water that is deficient can drain the metal's attempts to feed its "child," leading to lung and colon symptoms. In any case, your practitioner will use one or more components of the Eightfold Path Toward Health to bring your body back into balance, starting, perhaps, with a *qi gong* exercise system such as *tai chi*.

## *"Grand Ultimate Boxing"—the Art of* Tai Chi

Despite this common original translation, *tai chi* is not only a form of martial art and self-defense but also a system of exercises designed to balance the body and move energy through the meridians. Thousands of people, young and old alike, practice *tai chi* in China, here in the United States, and around the world. Walk through a park in New York, San Francisco, or Beijing any morning and you're sure to see a solitary figure or a group of enthusiasts practicing slow, graceful movements, seemingly led by an inner strength and concentration.

More than a dozen forms of *tai chi* are practiced, each centering on a different aspect of the art, such as exercise, meditation, self-defense, or the promotion of basic good health. No matter its focus, if you practice the art of *tai chi*, you'll almost certainly improve your coordination, balance, and body awareness. The practice will help calm your mind and reduce your emotional and psychological stress levels. You'll also improve your body alignment and posture, which will help reduce the physical stress placed on muscles and joints throughout the body.

The basic *qi gong* posture, common to *tai chi* and other energy exercises, is discussed in Chapter 6. It comprises standing with the feet apart, knees slightly bent, back straight, and arms held in front of the body; now imagine that you are holding a ball of *qi* in front of you while you maintain this posture for a few minutes. Doing so will help improve your circulation, relax you, and bring the body back into balance.

If you're interested in exploring the meditative and therapeutic effects of this ancient form of exercise, it's advisable to study with an experienced *tai chi* instructor. Ask your acupuncturist for suggestions. In the meantime, here are a few other simple *qi gong* exercises to try:

• *Walking on* qi Slowly walk in place by raising your left arm as you raise your right leg and then raising the opposite pair. Imagine yourself walking on a cloud of *qi*, light as a feather.

• *Flying* qi Stand erect, shoulders back but relaxed, with your palms facing each other. Move your hands slowly in a figure eight in front of your body. Your hands are like a bird's wings, floating through the air.

• *Turning* qi Twirl back and forth, allowing your arms to flap freely. This movement stimulates the *qi* to swirl around you, as if you were in the middle of a vortex of energy.

• *Build kidney* qi Ball your hands into fists and massage your back under the ribs so that it warms the back area. Quietly repeat the sound "tsh-oo-ee." You will feel the area over your kidneys warming. This warmth also strengthens the kidney energy.

## Treating Impotence

Since the water element reflects and controls sexual potency, when water energy is out of balance, problems with sexual functioning may arise. In the West, impotence—defined as a persistent inability to obtain an erection or to keep it long enough for sexual intercourse—is considered a complicated disorder involving hormonal, neurological, psychological, and vascular processes. An estimated half of all cases have psychological causes, including stress and anxiety. The other half of cases can be traced to physical problems, particularly cardiovascular disorders, diabetic nerve damage, or hormone disorders. Treatment depends on the underlying cause of the problem and may include one or more medications and/or psychological counseling.

Acupuncture, particularly in combination with conventional treatment, may prove useful in treating impotence. In a study published in a 1994 issue of *European Urology*, twenty of twenty-nine patients with a history of impotence were able to achieve erections after a varying number of acupuncture sessions. One reason for the success of this form of treatment is that acupuncture helps the body relax and dissipates stress, a definite plus no matter what the underlying problem. There is some evidence as well that acupuncture helps restore the appropriate balance of hormones related to the sexual response, including ACTH, testosterone, cortisol, LH (luteinizing hormone), and FSH (follicle-stimulating hormone). Some studies also indicate that acupuncture causes an increase in blood flow and improvement in nerve function, which goes to the heart of the two most common causes of physical impotency: cardiovascular problems and diabetic neuropathy.

## Treating Urinary Tract Problems

As the kidneys are an organ of the water element, kidney and bladder problems arise when this element is out of balance. Acupuncture appears to help treat such conditions as prostatitis (inflammation of the prostate gland), urinary incontinence (inability to hold urine), and nocturnal enuresis (bed-wetting). A Japanese study published in *Acta Urological Japonica* in 1994 followed seventeen patients with severe prostatitis. All seventeen patients experienced improvement, with 30 percent able to stop medication almost immediately.

Since prostatitis is an inflammation, it implies stagnation in the pelvis, which is governed by the kidneys. Other bladder and urinary conditions can occur when there is weakness and deficiency of the water channels. The treatment usually involves strengthening the appropriate channels. For instance, 85 percent of women treated for urinary burning and excessive frequency of urination were helped by acupuncture, according to a 1988 *Journal of Urology* study. In another instance, acupuncture aided children with enuresis by relaxing the bladder spasms causing their condition.

## *Treating Arthritis*

Within the Chinese medical paradigm, the kidneys are the deepest internal organ, and one of the kidneys' roles is to control the health of the bones. To have strong bones means to be solid internally, to feel secure, and that sense of strength and security derives from the water element. If water energy is blocked or unbalanced, bones and joints become weak.

In the West, conditions involving pain and dysfunction of the joints are often lumped under the general heading of arthritis, which is a blanket term for more than a dozen conditions affecting the joints. The two primary categories of arthritis are rheumatoid arthritis and osteoarthritis.

Rheumatoid arthritis is thought to be an autoimmune disease, in which the body's immune system attacks certain cells and organs. The joints of someone with this condition become swollen and red, and muscle, ligament, and bone tissue begins to erode. In some patients, rheumatoid arthritis affects not only one or more joints but also the heart, lungs, and eyes. Doctors treat rheumatoid arthritis with anti-inflammatory medicine, including both aspirin and corticosteroid drugs such as prednisone. Because this type of arthritis involves an inflammatory process, Chinese medicine treats it as stagnation of energy. Acupuncturists needle certain points in order to lessen this "stuckness." As noted in Chapter 5, stuckness and pain in the joints have a special name in Chinese medicine: bi syndrome.

Osteoarthritis is the most common form of joint disease. Although the precise mechanisms are unknown, it is clear that wear and tear is a principal cause. The cartilage that usually cushions the impact on the joint gradually deteriorates, leaving the joint vulnerable to pain and inflammation. Treatment with aspirin and corticosteroids is typical with this type of arthritis as well. However, the acupuncture treatment is very different from that performed on people with rheumatoid arthritis; it is directed more to strengthening and warming the water and associated channels.

Acupuncture may prove to be an effective treatment for the pain and disability related to both types of arthritis. A meta-analysis of several studies, published in a 1997 issue of the *Scandinavian Journal of Rheumatology*, and another study published in 1999 in *Rheumatology* show that acupuncture alleviates the pain of osteoarthritis, especially in combination with conventional treatments. Earlier, in 1985, a meta-analysis of several studies of the effects of acupuncture on rheumatoid arthritis led investigators to believe that acupuncture may have anti-inflammatory effects that reduce pain in rheumatoid arthritis patients.

## Treating Gynecological Conditions: Menopause and Infertility

Menopause is another condition that can be associated with kidney energy depletion, particularly the *yin* aspect of the kidneys. In this case, the decreasing levels of estrogens and the resulting cessation of menstrual periods are associated with a lack of the cooling, moistening aspect of a woman's body. Symptoms of menopause include hot flashes, dryness of the skin, and lack of secretions. Frequently, a restless fatigue and insomnia occur, which in Chinese medicine is the lack of rootedness and reserves.

Here in the West, of course, menopause is seen as part of the normal aging process that leads, inevitably, to the failure of the body to produce the proper balance of hormones responsible for menstruation and reproduction. These hormones include GnRH (gonadotropin-releasing hormone), LH, FSH, estrogen, and progesterone, each of which plays a specific role in the menstrual cycle.

In the West, infertility is considered a complicated problem with many potential underlying hormonal and physical causes. Chinese medicine also considers infertility to be the end result of several types of imbalances. As with other conditions, there can be stuckness and block-age in the pelvic area, leading to a lack of proper cycling and even phys-ical problems with the uterus and fallopian tubes (the tubes that connect the ovaries to the uterus). Other instances can be characterized by defi-ciency of heat in the pelvis, or a general lack of blood and energy. Many times, a practitioner of Chinese medicine will use a combination of acu-puncture, moxibustion, and herbal medicine to correct the imbalance.

Surprisingly few studies have been done on the effects of acupunc-ture on menopausal symptoms, but anecdotal evidence points to its effi-cacy, especially in alleviating hot flashes and other side effects of the loss of hormones. Infertility studies are more common, and many, including a 1997 study published in *Acupuncture and Electro-Therapeutics Research*, indicate that acupuncture could help trigger the proper release of GnRH and FSH, thereby correcting a hormone imbalance and allowing conception to occur.

## Using Acupuncture to Rebalance Water Energy

An acupuncturist chooses from several points along the kidney and bladder channels in treating a water energy imbalance. Among the most common are the following:

• *Kidney 3 ("greater mountain stream")* For water energy to be strong, it must flow steadily and smoothly. Acupuncturists frequently use this source point on the kidney channel to facilitate the flow. The point is useful in combination with others in treating fatigue, menopausal symp-toms, and other dry and hot conditions. The point is behind the medial anklebone.

• *Kidney 24 ("spirit burial ground")* This point is on the chest, next to the breastbone. As its familiar name implies, acupuncturists needle it when they notice that a patient's spirit is flickering and needs to be rekindled. It is a powerful point, and though used sparingly, its results can be profound. Although this point is on the kidney channel and draws from the depths of the water element, it pertains to the spirit in any element.

• *Bladder 10 ("heavenly pillar")* This point is on the back of the head where the large muscle of the neck joins the head. It is a "window to the sky" point, which means it opens up the bladder channel to the possibilities of infinite reserves and energy. Because of its location, it can be used for structural problems as well.

• *Bladder 23 ("kidney correspondence")* There are back *shu* points (also called associated effect points) on the bladder channel that actually address problems with the meridian for which they are named. Found on the lumbar area near the adrenal glands, this point is used to strengthen reserves, support the will, and generally address kidney energy problems. Acupuncturists tend to use moxa on this point.

• *Governing Vessel 4 ("gate of life")* This point is on the spine at the same level as the "kidney correspondence" point. Although not technically a water point, it is here that the drive and strength that characterize the water element can be marshalled. Acupuncturists also use it to treat physical problems in the spine, such as arthritis, as well as behavior problems involving weakness or lack of courage—behavior we might call "spineless."

## Maintaining Water Energy Balance

When one's water energy is depleted, fear and anxiety result. With no reserves, one can feel like a person caught in a flood, with nothing solid to cling to, no "piece of the rock." Fortunately, there are ways that even people with deficient *jing* (the ancestral life force stored in the kidneys) can increase their reserves. And the more we build our day-to-day reserves, the less we have to use up our *jing* throughout life. In Chinese medicine, having plentiful *jing* means being able to stay active and healthy and maintain a youthful vibrancy into an advanced age. Building *jing* involves living a healthful lifestyle.

Specifically, energy from the food we eat and the air we breathe helps to maintain and build our day-to-day reserves. A healthy diet of fresh, whole foods will provide maximum benefit, while a diet that damages the body, such as one loaded with fat, grease, coffee, alcohol, and refined foods, will deplete the reserves. Lack of sleep, an imbalance between activity and rest, will also act to drain the body's reserves. Here are measures you can take to build *jing*:

• *Meditate!* People with limited water reserves can become irritable, uneasy, and anxious when their energy is thrown off balance, and there's perhaps no better way to maintain focus and serenity than performing a meditation practice on a regular basis, preferably daily. If you're a water type, meditation will also appeal to your philosophical and spiritual side, allowing you to explore and revel in your naturally self-reflective nature. Chapter 6 provides more information on meditation and meditation techniques, and your practitioner will also be able to offer suggestions on getting started.

• *Take herbs to build your reserves* The core of most kidney herbal formulas, both *yin* and *yang*, is a famous formula called *liu wei di huang wan* (six flavor rehmannia). The herbs in this formula work to solidify and moisten the kidney *qi*. If the kidney *yang* is deficient, warming herbs are added. If there is some inflammation stemming from a lack of fluids, heat-reducing herbs are added. Potency and male sexual function necessitate both kidney *yin* and *yang* strength. Sometimes, the skin of geckos or other fast-moving lizards is used in these formulas (though, in Western cultures, the thought of boiled lizard is far from an aphrodisiac!). Your acupuncturist will help find the right herbs to keep your water element strong and in balance.

• *Get enough sleep* Americans get significantly less sleep than they did a generation ago. To make matters worse, the afternoon catnap has gone the way of the ten-cent hot dog, and even when we lie in bed, our minds are frequently filled with thoughts of what we haven't done. Without sleep, we cannot restore our system to its full reserve. Remember that we need *yin* to balance all of the *yang* in our lives.

• *Drink lots of water* Nourishing your body by drinking at least six to eight glasses of water per day is especially important for someone with strong water energy. The fact that we tend to live and work in closed, heated, and dry environments only adds to the need. Without sufficient fluid in the body, kidney reserves become low. Stiff joints, fatigue, and even confused mental function may improve with proper hydration.

• *Exercise, exercise, exercise!* Because people have a tendency to suffer from joint and bone diseases when their water energy becomes imbalanced, it's essential to perform both stretching exercises to keep the body flexible and weight-bearing exercises to help build and maintain bone tissue. Ample data support the preventive effects of exercise on osteoporosis, osteoarthritis, and even chronic fatigue and fibromyalgia syndromes. In addition, the best way to become strong and develop energy reserves is to get in shape. If exercise isn't currently part of your daily routine, walk straight to your nearest gym or fitness center and get started!

PART III

# HOW ACUPUNCTURE CAN WORK FOR YOU

Most experts agree that the future of medicine lies in an integration of Eastern and Western philosophies and techniques. This final section shows you how to make acupuncture part of your health-care plan, with information about insurance and choosing the right practitioner for you. It offers an optimistic but realistic view of a future of truly integrative medicine, in which the best of both approaches work together to bring health and balance to body and mind.

10

# INTEGRATING ACUPUNCTURE

EARLIER CHAPTERS OF THIS BOOK spelled out the differences between Eastern and Western medicine and the challenges these differences present in attempting to integrate acupuncture into conventional Western medicine. This chapter features the progress that's been made in those efforts and the state of acupuncture today, at the start of the twenty-first century.

## Where and How Acupuncture Is Used in the United States Today

As much as one may bemoan the battles that remain to be fought in integrating acupuncture with conventional Western medicine, it is nonetheless necessary to recognize the tremendous strides made in the three decades or so since journalist James Reston chronicled for American readers his observations of acupuncture in action on a trip to China. After thirty years, acupuncture has established itself in mainstream America. What was once unfamiliar to most doctors, even as a word, now has two defined treatment codes in the American Medical Association's bible for physicians, *Physician's Current Procedural Terminology*.

But it was the National Institutes of Health's landmark Scientific Consensus Conference Report on acupuncture in 1997 that turned the tide of acceptance, particularly among physicians. The NIH had convened a panel of twelve members representing multiple fields of medicine and acupuncture to hear evidence about acupuncture's effectiveness and to issue a statement of findings based on its conclusions. The panel identified three conditions (postoperative and chemotherapy nausea and vomiting, nausea and vomiting of pregnancy, and postoperative dental pain) in which it determined that acupuncture treatment is clearly effective. It also identified a dozen or so additional chronic conditions and pain syndromes for which panel members felt there was compelling, but not overwhelming, evidence of acupuncture's effectiveness. (Note that the World Health Organization identifies forty conditions for which acupuncture is an approved treatment.) Through its National Center for Complementary and Alternative Medicine (NCCAM), the NIH continues to support and fund research and studies of acupuncture and other complementary therapies, intent on establishing clinical criteria that meet Western medicine standards.

As of early 2001, twenty-one government-sponsored trials looking at acupuncture in a variety of conditions were under way. Some of these conditions, such as hypertension, cerebral palsy in children, and sinusitis in HIV patients, have not been studied before. Others, such as fibromyalgia, osteoarthritis, and depression, have had inconclusive studies performed in the past. One current study includes acupuncture along with drug therapies as alternatives to hormonal therapy for patients who have had breast cancer. Another will look at the cost-effectiveness of using acupuncture to treat osteoarthritis of the knee, which costs the United States millions of dollars each year.

The NIH panel's findings were consistent with the beliefs of many Americans. The Food and Drug Administration (FDA) reported that in 1993 Americans had received an estimated 12 million acupuncture treatments. And a 1998 survey reported in the *Journal of the American Medical Association* found that more than 42 percent of Americans—83 million of them—had used some form of complementary medicine the previous year, paying more than $27 billion out-of-pocket for the privilege that many hope will soon be a right. This dollar figure is especially significant when you consider that this amount exceeded spending for *hospital* services not covered by health insurance.

While most acupuncture treatments still take place in the offices of acupuncturists, an exciting and promising integration of acupuncture into conventional Western medical practice is occurring in a variety of health-care environments. Some of America's most prestigious health-care centers are exploring the potential of complementary treatments. Key among them are the following programs:

• Beth Israel Medical Center in New York City opened its $5 million Center for Health and Healing in 2000. Physicians and nurses work in collaboration with acupuncturists and other practitioners of complementary medicine to provide integrative health-care services for patients who desire them.

• Cedars-Sinai Medical Center in Los Angeles conducted a pilot study in which open-heart surgery patients received acupuncture treatments following the surgery. Ninety-five percent (nineteen of twenty) reported that the treatments significantly improved their recoveries, leading Cedars-Sinai to expand the study to include more patients as well as a control group.

• More than eight hundred drug-dependency programs in twenty states incorporate acupuncture into their models. In Dade County, Florida, first-time offenders are given a choice of jail or an acupuncture and counseling program. Patients who complete these programs have lower rearrest rates on drug-related charges than those not treated with the acupuncture and counseling program.

There are almost fifteen thousand licensed acupuncturists in the United States and at least half as many medical (physician) acupuncturists. Most medical students are exposed to various complementary therapies, and some take introductory classes in these subjects. For example, the acupuncture training program affiliated with the University of California–Los Angeles School of Medicine provides an overview of acupuncture theories and practices and has experienced steadily increasing enrollment since its inception.

Residents in family practice at Lutheran General Hospital in Park Ridge, Illinois, now have the option of completing a one-month rotation in the hospital's Center for Complementary Medicine. The training begins in a way few other rotations can: with new doctors receiving complementary therapies to treat problems of their own that they identify to Center practitioners. This gives them a personalized taste of complementary medicine and, it is hoped, a lasting positive impression as well.

The University of Arizona School of Medicine has established a fellowship program for physicians who are interested in specializing in the burgeoning field of integrative medicine. These physicians, already board-certified in a specialty such as family practice or internal medicine, spend two years developing expertise in a complementary field such as acupuncture or homeopathy.

## Who Pays for Acupuncture Treatments?

The short answer to the question of who pays is . . . you do. While the NCCAM estimates that nearly 80 percent of health insurers currently offer some level of coverage for acupuncture treatments, most coverage is so limited that patients still pay for the majority of acupuncture costs.

The exception is for acupuncture treatments provided by a physician (M.D. or D.O.) for conditions that the insurer identifies as appropriate for acupuncture, such as migraine, back pain, and trigeminal neuralgia, among others.

At the time of this writing, six states require insurers to offer coverage for complementary treatments as part of their overall benefits packages, and more are likely to follow suit in the near future. One strategy recently adopted by insurance companies is setting up so-called affinity programs, through which they enlist acupuncturists to accept lower fees from the company's patients. The company then advertises to its subscribers that they have acupuncture as a benefit. The "benefit" is the list of acupuncturists that accept lower fees.

In Washington, insurers filed suit to overturn the state law mandating coverage for complementary therapies. They even brought the issue before the U.S. Supreme Court, which declined to hear it, leaving the mandated coverage requirements intact. This was a significant victory for patients, which had been closely watched by providers and insurers alike. Industry insiders expect other states to follow Washington's lead, though it's anybody's guess how long it might take for mandated coverage for complementary treatments to become the national standard.

Insurers insist that forcing them to cover complementary therapies will cause premiums to rise, but so far there is little evidence to support this contention. In fact, acupuncture often replaces more costly treatments such as medications and physical therapy and also helps people to heal faster than they would with conventional medical care. In the long run, it's more likely that regular use of acupuncture will reduce what insurers call utilization—the amount of health-care services that insured patients use. This should lower, not raise, premiums, since it will contribute to lower costs for insurance companies.

Some information on the cost savings associated with acupuncture is already available. One study of six clinics in five states looked at efficacy and cost savings of acupuncture. Of the patients treated with acupuncture, 91.5 percent reported disappearance or improvement of symptoms; 84 percent said they saw their M.D.s less; 79 percent said they used fewer prescription drugs; and 70 percent of those to whom surgery had been recommended said they avoided the surgery. In addition, a controlled clinical trial evaluated the use of acupuncture combined with standard stroke protocol for the treatment of paralysis due to stroke. Effective or markedly effective results were found for more than 80 percent of the patients receiving acupuncture, with a cost savings of $26,000 per patient.

However, until more of the proper cost-effectiveness studies are performed, there will be a reluctance on the part of insurance plans, and by conventional medical doctors, to accept acupuncture. In the words of a physician representative of Blue Cross speaking at a recent conference, "Increasingly, coverage is dependent on evidence of clinical effectiveness. . . . In the private sector, preferred provider organizations and health maintenance organizations increasingly rely on scientific evidence of improved health outcomes as a basis for making positive coverage decisions." It is this increasing reliance on clinical studies (termed evidence-based medicine) that will determine how effectively acupuncture will be incorporated into mainstream medicine in the twenty-first century.

If you are in a group health insurance plan that does not cover acupuncture and other complementary treatments, tell your human resources department or union representative that you would like to see it added. It often doesn't cost employers much to add this benefit, and insurers know that dissatisfied consumers will take their business elsewhere. You should find support for your position among your coworkers: one New York study showed that 13 percent of respondents had used acupuncture, and 80 percent of those people described their experience as favorable. Nationwide, people make more than 20 million visits to acupuncturists each year.

Though traditional health insurance coverage is convenient, it isn't the only option for getting acupuncture treatments paid for. If you work for an employer that offers flexible spending accounts, you could end up having nearly all of your acupuncture expenses, up to the account's annual limit, reimbursed. A flexible spending account allows you to contribute pretax dollars from your salary to a holding fund. You can then receive reimbursement for eligible out-of-pocket expenses. The catchword here is "eligible." Flexible spending accounts have different criteria, so be sure to check with your company's human resources department about yours. Because flexible spending accounts divert a portion of your income before you pay taxes on it, the Internal Revenue Service sets the annual contribution limits. In 2001, the maximum contribution was $5,000.

## How Much Do Acupuncture Treatments Cost?

As is the case with most other services, fees for acupuncture treatments vary among geographic and population regions. An initial consultation might cost $100 or more, with subsequent treatments averaging from $30 to $80 each. A course of treatment might run from several days for an acute problem to several weeks for chronic conditions. A survey of clinical studies indicated that a minimum of six to eight treatments resulted in more success with pain conditions, while at least ten treatments and sometimes as many as twenty-five were necessary in medical conditions such as asthma.

Physician acupuncturists typically charge more than nonphysician acupuncturists, though health insurance is more likely to cover treatments by a physician acupuncturist. Always ask your acupuncturist at the onset of treatment how long the course of treatment will last and what it will cost. As with any health treatment, beware of those who guarantee success. No one can predict the future, and no treatment always works perfectly for everyone.

## Acupuncturist Qualifications

Forty-two states do not separately regulate the training and practice of acupuncture by physicians (M.D.s and D.O.s), allowing them to practice acupuncture within the scope of their licenses to practice medicine. Some of these states also include chiropractors, naturopaths, dentists, or podiatrists in this definition and may or may not require additional training. A few states have laws restricting the practice of acupuncture to persons licensed to practice medicine. Most states regulate non-physician acupuncturists, though standards and requirements vary widely.

Though Louisiana regulates the practice of acupuncture, it does not have an examination. Two states, Kansas and Michigan, do not have laws regulating the practice of acupuncture, but allow acupuncturists to practice through a ruling by the state board of medical examiners. Michigan's attorney general has ruled that acupuncture is a certified medical procedure and is regulated accordingly (and also has legislation pending). In addition to Michigan, states in which regulatory legislation is pending include Alabama, Kentucky, Oklahoma, and Wyoming. Though certification of acupuncturists is a state-by-state process, most states require that an acupuncturist graduate from an accredited school and pass the National Council for the Accreditation of Acupuncturists examination (California and Nevada have their own examinations).

The currently accepted training program for an acupuncturist takes three years to complete, after which the student receives a master's degree. In addition, some schools offer training in Eastern medicine, a four-year program that includes acupuncture, herbs, and massage techniques. Currently, forty U.S. schools either are accredited or are candidates for accreditation in the granting of acupuncture degrees. The

## STATES THAT REGULATE THE PRACTICE OF ACUPUNCTURE

| | | |
|---|---|---|
| Alaska | Louisiana | Ohio |
| Arizona | Maine | Oregon |
| Arkansas | Maryland | Pennsylvania |
| California | Massachusetts | Rhode Island |
| Colorado | Minnesota | South Carolina |
| Connecticut | Missouri | Tennessee |
| District of Columbia | Montana | Texas |
| Florida | Nebraska | Utah |
| Georgia | Nevada | Vermont |
| Hawaii | New Hampshire | Virginia |
| Idaho | New Jersey | Washington |
| Illinois | New Mexico | West Virginia |
| Indiana | New York | Wisconsin |
| Iowa | North Carolina | |

accrediting body, the Accreditation Commission for Acupuncture and Oriental Medicine (ACAOM), is recognized by the U.S. Department of Education.

Accreditation helps to standardize training and education for acupuncturists. ACAOM accreditation for doctoral programs includes the following requirements:

- The institution or school must be accredited by the appropriate
  state or federal entities for higher education.
- The school must also offer a master's degree in acupuncture or
  Eastern medicine (accredited by ACAOM).
- The acupuncture program must have a minimum of four
  thousand hours of study for each doctorate student (in master's
  and doctoral programs combined), with twelve hundred of those
  hours at the doctorate level.
- The acupuncture program's administrator and teaching staff must
  be appropriately qualified.
- The curriculum must cover competencies in five key areas:
  advanced patient assessment and diagnosis, advanced clinical
  intervention and treatment, consultation and collaboration,
  clinical supervision and practice management, and clinical
  evaluation and research.

Some of the schools offer programs for physicians, chiropractors, and other practitioners who want to expand their knowledge and expertise. There are also several schools of naturopathy, culminating in a doctor of naturopathy degree. Acupuncture is within the scope of practice of many naturopaths in the states in which they are licensed.

The American Academy of Medical Acupuncture (AAMA) has established standardized criteria for physician acupuncturists. These include education and experience standards as well as proficiency and certification examinations. Most states as well as health insurance plans are beginning to recognize the AAMA as the credentialing organization for state licensing or registration, hospital privileges, and eligibility to participate in insurance payment or reimbursement programs. If your acupuncturist is a physician, he or she should be an AAMA member in good standing.

Acupuncture is, after all, a specialty practice. In 2000, the AAMA established a Board of Medical Acupuncture to certify physician acupuncturists in their specialty. To qualify for board certification, physician acupuncturists must pass the AAMA certification examination as well as complete three hundred hours of acupuncture study, including one hundred clinical hours; must have proficiency in at least two acupuncture systems (such as French energetics or the Five Elements); and must have performed at least five hundred acupuncture treatments in clinical practice. The goal of the AAMA is to create a recognized medical specialty.

Nonphysician acupuncturists may belong to the Acupuncture and Oriental Medicine Alliance, the American College of Acupuncture and Oriental Medicine, or one or more of the regional, state, and local organizations for acupuncturists.

# How to Find an Acupuncturist

The best way to find an acupuncturist is by word of mouth, either through referral by your doctor or through friends or family members. More and more, physicians are referring patients to acupuncturists. In a 1996 Kaiser study, published in the *Western Journal of Medicine* in 1998, 57.2 percent of the primary care physicians in Northern California said they had recommended acupuncture in the previous twelve months.

The websites of the organizations cited in this chapter also offer referrals (see the Appendix). Always check an acupuncturist's credentials, whether the practitioner is a physician or nonphysician. Ask to see evidence of completed training and required certification or licensing (if applicable in your state). Also ask about the acupuncturist's experience, areas of interest, and personal philosophies that guide the treatment approach. Most important in this era of potentially deadly infectious diseases, verify that the acupuncturist uses a new, freshly opened package of sterile, disposable needles for each treatment. (This is an FDA requirement.)

Don't be hesitant to meet with several acupuncturists before deciding on one to see for treatment. As with other care providers, an important element of treatment is the trust you have in the practitioner and the relationship that develops between the two of you. If you don't feel comfortable talking generally with the acupuncturist, you're certainly not going to be willing to share your feelings, fears, and personal information. Communication with any health provider is critical in the healing process. Let your intuition guide your decision; if something doesn't feel quite right, move on.

## What to Expect on Your First Visit

This is not your typical doctor's visit! The acupuncturist, whether a physician or not, will usually take thirty to sixty minutes to listen to you describe your symptoms, ask about your health history, and examine you. The extent of the questioning may take you aback, but remember that acupuncture theory involves who we are in all aspects of the body, mind, and spirit. You may be asked detailed questions about your bowel habits, or how you obtained the tiniest little scars (which may lie across acupuncture meridians), or even about your favorite season and foods.

While some aspects of the examination, such as palpation of your abdomen, will be familiar to you, others may come as a surprise. Don't be alarmed when your tongue receives more scrutiny than any other body part. In acupuncture, the tongue is the harbinger of the body's health and reflects day-to-day progress in treatment. No doubt, the pulse will also get a lot of attention, and you might be asked if certain points on your abdomen and elsewhere are tender. Your acupuncturist will likely spend some time examining your external ear as well.

Some offices have waiting rooms, but many acupuncturists work privately in small offices or have treatment rooms in their homes. You will usually first speak to the acupuncturist while you both are sitting in chairs, or with you sitting on the exam table, and then be asked to remove some of your clothing. Most acupuncturists need you to be at least partly undressed to reach all the points on the body, and they should have clean gowns available and a private changing area.

You will then probably be asked to lie facing up on the examination table. Some of the examination might be performed with you sitting. The room should be warm enough and the table comfortable; the average acupuncture treatment takes thirty to forty-five minutes. During the treatment, you may be lying faceup with needles in your limbs and/or abdomen. When points on the back are used, you may either lie facedown or sit up.

Some acupuncture systems involve leaving needles in, while other techniques remove the needles after a brief period; you then are left to lie quietly so that the energy can balance. Moxa is sometimes used in conjunction with needles. Moxa can be used in a lit "cigar" form to warm an area, placed on a needle and burned to warm its shaft, or placed on the body and briefly lit to warm an acupoint. The acupuncturist must know your complete medical history, as moxa and some needling should not be used in certain cases, such as application on the legs of a person with diabetes.

Perhaps the most common question that I am asked is whether acupuncture hurts. The honest answer is "yes and no." There definitely is a sensation when a needle hits the point, although there's hardly any pain when it actually penetrates skin. The sensation can feel like a cramp, like hitting the "funny bone" in the elbow, or sometimes like a minor electrical jolt. In fact, the Chinese language has four different words for *da qi*, the sensation of grabbing the *qi* with an acupuncture needle. The feeling dissipates whether the needle is left in or not, and most people do not find the sensation unpleasant.

Every once in a while, an acupuncture treatment has an immediate profound effect on a patient or symptom. More likely, you will feel relaxed, even dreamy. You may doze off on the treatment table, even with needles in. After the treatment, it's common to feel energized and calm. It's generally recommended that a patient not drink alcohol after a treatment, but there are typically no restrictions on exercising, driving, or other activities.

# What to Expect from Your Treatment Protocol

Don't expect a symptom to disappear immediately. Acupuncture treatments are more often cumulative. I ask patients to look back over several treatments and tell me if they can perceive the change over time. Sometimes, you might even feel a bit worse after the first few treatments. Of course, after eight or ten treatments (usually one or two treatments per week), you should be able to perceive enough of an effect to either continue treatment or stop.

Many patients experience positive effects that they did not expect. I have a patient who came to me because of headaches. Her headaches are only moderately better, but she says that the treatments have improved her ability to cope with the stresses of her workplace so much that she has continued treatment. Another patient who came for back pains found that her asthma improved when her back was treated. Others feel an emotional lift from treatment and notice the difference when they have not been treated in a while. Thus, it is possible to use acupuncture as a health maintenance system.

Acupuncture has clear effects beyond the day of treatment itself, but chronic problems can sometimes recur if the energy movement isn't reinforced. For this reason and others, an acupuncturist may recommend that a patient continue treatments on a less frequent basis than the more common weekly treatments. This may be once every two to four weeks, or once a season.

# Challenges for the Future

Despite the fervent hopes of many people, widespread acceptance of acupuncture in conventional Western medicine will not come without challenge. A major stumbling block for many conventional physicians is the issue of clinical study results (see Chapter 3). Although the NCCAM funds numerous studies at respected medical centers throughout the United States, it's not always possible to conduct the studies according to traditional standards. How, for example, does a researcher "fake" acupuncture treatments for a placebo group? It is hoped that efforts to establish a "placebo needle" will solve this problem.

Western research operates in a different paradigm from that of Eastern practice. While the Western way defines results in terms of time ("we'll study this for two years"), the Eastern model considers time in terms of results (treatment is effective when it relieves symptoms and restores health). Though acupuncture is a good start in building a bridge between these opposing paradigms, it's not likely to resolve their fundamental differences until Western researchers and practitioners can look beyond what they hold to be truths.

This is not to say there is no hope for more comprehensive integration of acupuncture into conventional Western medical treatments. To the contrary, there is more hope than ever that this integration is on the horizon. After all, when you consider that it's taken twenty-five hundred years for acupuncture to evolve to its current practice, the thirty years spent trying to spread the word seem but a flash in time. If there is a lesson to be learned from the past three decades of experience, it is that Western patients and physicians alike are opening themselves to the possibilities that Eastern medicine offers. Change does not come easily, and Western practitioners have long struggled to maintain standards of practice that put the patient's best interests first. It's now time for them to recognize and accept that doing so sometimes means trusting in methods that defy an easy explanation in Western terms.

# AFTERWORD
## The Future of Medicine

As he sits waiting for his doctor, a man considers his discomfort. When the doctor beckons him into the examination room, he already feels better, physically and emotionally, as he notices the doctor's careful gaze and feels her gentle, reassuring touch as she helps him onto the table. He knows he has time to tell his doctor about his symptoms, and he proceeds to do so: his stomach burns, his muscles ache, and his sinuses persistently drip. He is driven to tell his doctor every detail of every symptom, and he waits for the comfort and sympathy he needs so desperately. The doctor knows that her patient has this need for attention, and she is glad she is no longer so burdened by bureaucratic imperatives that she has to shoo him out of the office in ten or fifteen minutes.

Although the doctor is not an acupuncturist, she received training in Eastern techniques and philosophy in medical school. She now recognizes when energy is out of balance and notes that this patient could be exhibiting symptoms of earth imbalance. She questions him about his symptoms and conducts a full physical examination. She orders tests to evaluate his stomach problem, including a blood test and an x-ray of the stomach. She also does blood testing to evaluate the muscle aches, although it is her impression that this is not a disease, but rather the kind of muscle aches associated with lack of regular exercise. Finally, she determines that the patient's sinuses are inflamed but not infected.

The patient is surprised by several aspects of this visit. He is pleased by the amount of time the doctor spent with him and curious about the great amount of physical touching that took place during the examination. Some of the questions about his lifestyle and daily habits seemed out of the ordinary, but so far, the results of his interactions with the doctor and the treatment of other ailments have left him feeling in more control of his health, and healthier, than he has for a long time.

At the end of the visit, the doctor prescribes two treatments for his stomach ailment: an herbal remedy and a conventional pharmaceutical medication in case the herbs fail to solve the problem. She also makes some lifestyle suggestions designed to alleviate his sinus drip, including running a humidifier in his bedroom every night and using a prescribed nasal inhaler. Finally, she refers the patient to an acupuncturist, explaining that she believes his symptoms are caused by an internal imbalance of energy that an acupuncturist is trained to resolve.

The doctor gives the acupuncturist a call before her patient's appointment. She tells the acupuncturist that she believes her patient has a dampness condition affecting the earth channels. She also notifies the patient's health maintenance organization (HMO) that she has referred the patient to an acupuncturist for dampness in the earth channels, leading to stomach problems (which she is still in the process of diagnosing medically), myalgia (the medical term for muscle aches), and sinusitis. The HMO notifies her that it will allow twelve visits, plus the initial visit, with the acupuncturist.

When the patient arrives at his first appointment with the acupuncturist, he's again surprised at the time and care this health professional devotes to him. The acupuncturist takes a complete history, including questions about the patient's upbringing, his relationships, his favorite activities, and his diet. He looks at the patient's tongue, palpates the muscles, spends a long time on the pulse, and pokes several places on the abdomen, feeling the temperature as well. Then, he talks to the patient about earth energy and the possible results of treatment. The acupuncture treatments begin later that week. Needles are used on the back and abdomen, as well as on the feet and along the lower legs. The herb moxa is used to heat some of the needles.

Shortly after the second treatment, the patient feels oddly energized. On suggestion from the acupuncturist, he begins a regimen of exercise by taking a twenty-minute walk each morning. He also avoids eating salads and other cold foods, as well as sweets, as these foods tend to exacerbate an earth energy imbalance.

By the third treatment, the patient's stomachache has subsided, and he never has to take the prescription medicine. The patient has his treatments faithfully, once per week, and by the second month, he has developed the habit of taking his dog for a long walk each morning. His muscle aches are gone. He has lost several extra pounds, and he feels mentally and physically more vital. The acupuncturist focuses some treatments on the sinuses, using points on the face and scalp, as well as the abdomen. The patient notices that his sinuses are clearer for several days after each treatment.

By the time he visits his conventional doctor again, he's a changed man. His symptoms have nearly subsided 100 percent, and he uses the inhaler for his sinuses only occasionally. What's more, he seems—and feels—less needy, answering the doctor's questions without excessive detail or the need for sympathy.

The doctor smiles. She remembers a time when acupuncture was not a common part of a doctor's skills, when she did not understand how to recognize energy and its imbalances, when she was not trained to address her patients in a holistic manner. She remembers when insurance companies didn't recognize the value of Chinese medicine in treating common conditions and in saving money. And she recalls when the population considered acupuncture to be something strange and exotic, rather than the safe and useful treatment system that it is today. She is glad that things have changed, so she smiles. And so does her patient.

# APPENDIX
## Resources for
## More Information

If you're interested in finding out more about acupuncture or in studying acupuncture yourself, contact any of the national organizations listed here, which offer information about both acupuncture and Chinese medicine in the United States.

*Accreditation Commission for Acupuncture and Oriental Medicine (ACAOM)*
1010 Wayne Avenue, Suite 1270
Silver Spring, MD 20910
(301) 608-9680; fax (301) 608-9576

Established in June 1982, the Accreditation Commission acts as an independent body to evaluate professional master's degree and professional master's-level certificate and diploma programs in acupuncture and in Eastern medicine with concentrations in both acupuncture and herbal therapy. The standard is a level of performance, integrity, and quality that merits the confidence of the educational community and the public.

*Acupuncture and Oriental Medicine Alliance*
14637 Starr Road S.E.
Olalla, WA 98359
(253) 851-6896; fax (253) 851-6883
www.acupuncturealliance.org

The Acupuncture Alliance is a national professional membership
association founded to represent the diversity of practitioners of
acupuncture and Chinese medicine in the United States. The
Alliance is committed to integrating acupuncture and Chinese
medicine into the American health-care system as well as
fostering high-quality health care, education, and research.

*American Academy of Medical Acupuncture (AAMA)*
5820 Wilshire Boulevard, Suite 500
Los Angeles, CA 90036
(323) 937-5514
www.medicalacupuncture.org

The purpose of the AAMA is to promote the integration of
concepts from traditional and modern forms of acupuncture into
Western medical training and thereby synthesize a more
comprehensive approach to health care.

*American College of Acupuncture and Oriental Medicine*
9100 Park West Drive
Houston, TX 77063
(800) 729-4456, (713) 780-9777; fax (713) 781-5781
www.acaom.edu

The primary goal of the American College of Acupuncture and
Oriental Medicine is to train health-care practitioners in the
diagnosis and treatment of health problems based on the theories
and principles of acupuncture and Eastern medicine.

### Council of Colleges of Acupuncture and Oriental Medicine (CCAOM)

1010 Wayne Avenue, Suite 1270
Silver Spring, MD 20910
(301) 608-9175; fax (301) 608-9576
www.ccaom.org

Formed in 1982 for the purpose of advancing the status of acupuncture and Eastern medicine in the United States, the CCAOM has developed academic and clinical guidelines and core curriculum requirements for master's-level and doctoral-level programs in acupuncture and Chinese medicine.

### National Certification Commission for Acupuncture and Oriental Medicine (NCCAOM)

11 Canal Center Plaza, Suite 300
Alexandria, VA 22314
(703) 548-9004; fax (703) 548-9079
www.nccaom.org

The NCCAOM, formerly known as the National Commission for the Certification of Acupuncturists, was established by the profession in 1982 to promote nationally recognized standards of competence for acupuncture and Eastern medicine. The NCCAOM has certified more than five thousand individuals in acupuncture and one thousand in Chinese herbology. NCCAOM certification is used as the basis for licensure in 90 percent of the states that have set standards of practice for acupuncture.

*National Center for Complementary and Alternative Medicine
(NCCAM)*
P.O. Box 8218
Silver Spring, MD 20907-8218
1-888-644-6226; fax (301) 495-4957
http://nccam. nih.gov

The NCCAM, a division of the National Institutes of Health, was
established by Congress in 1998 to develop and support research
on complementary and alternative medicine. Its primary mission is
to provide the public with acurate information about the safety
and effectiveness of alternative therapies.

# INDEX

# ABOUT THE AUTHOR

GLENN S. ROTHFELD, M.D., M.AC., has been in the forefront of the complementary medicine movement for the past twenty-five years. A former Clinical Fellow of Harvard University School of Medicine's Channing Laboratory, he is currently Clinical Assistant Professor of family medicine at Tufts University School of Medicine, where he developed one of the nation's first courses on alternative medicine. Dr. Rothfeld was trained in acupuncture at the Traditional Acupuncture Institute in Columbia, Maryland, and furthered his studies at the College of Traditional Chinese Acupuncture in Leamington Spa, England. He is a frequent lecturer, and has authored six prior books on complementary medicine topics. He is currently medical director of Whole-Health New England, a complementary medicine center in Arlington, Massachusetts (*www.WholeHealthNE.com*). He lives in Lexington, Massachusetts, with his wife and children.